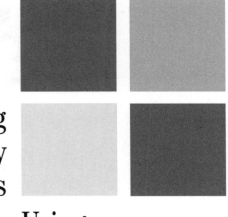

Compensating for Memory Deficits

Using a Systematic Approach

Compensating for Memory Deficits

Using a Systematic Approach

Susan K. Kime, OTR/L

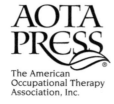

AOTA PRESS

The American
Occupational Therapy
Association, Inc.

Vision Statement

The American Occupational Therapy Association advances occupational therapy as the pre-eminent profession in promoting the health, productivity, and quality of life of individuals and society through the therapeutic application of occupation.

Mission Statement

The American Occupational Therapy Association advances the quality, availability, use, and support of occupational therapy through standard-setting, advocacy, education, and research on behalf of its members and the public.

AOTA Staff

Frederick P. Somers, Executive Director
Christopher M. Bluhm, Chief Operating Officer
Audrey Rothstein, Director, Marketing and Communications

Chris Davis, Managing Editor, AOTA Press
Barbara Dickson, Production Editor

Robert A. Sacheli, Manager, Creative Services
Sarah E. Ely, Book Production Coordinator

Marge Wasson, Marketing Manager
Elizabeth Johnson, Marketing Specialist

The American Occupational Therapy Association, Inc.
4720 Montgomery Lane
Bethesda, MD 20814
Phone: 301-652-AOTA (2682)
TDD: 800-377-8555
Fax: 301-652-7711
www.aota.org
To order: 1-877-404-AOTA (2682)

ISBN: 1-56900-219-3

Library of Congress Control Number: 2006923122

Design by Sarah E. Ely
Composition by The Electronic Quill, Silver Spring, Maryland
Printed by Versa Press, Inc., East Peoria, Illinois

Contents

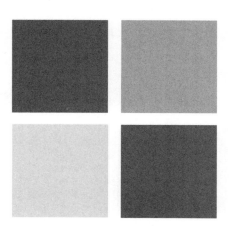

List of Figures

Foreword

It is with great pleasure that I write in support of this book written by a very imaginative and creative occupational therapist. I had the pleasure of working with Susan Kime for 3 months in Arizona in 1993 at the Barrow Neurological Unit, St. Joseph's Hospital, when I was on sabbatical there with Dr. George Prigatano. So impressed was I by her practical solutions and clinical skills in helping people compensate for cognitive difficulties following brain injury that I invited her to come to the United Kingdom to help train our staff before the opening of the Oliver Zangwill Center in 1996.

People with memory deficits following nonprogressive brain injury are very unlikely to regain their premorbid level of memory functioning once the phase of natural recovery is over. To optimize their level of independence in the everyday world in which they are to live, we need to help them compensate for their memory problems. However, memory problems do not exist in a vacuum. The emotional consequences of cognitive impairment and brain injury will affect how people respond to treatment. Level of insight and degree of awareness in the individual will influence progress in rehabilitation, as will the amount and nature of the support provided by family members and the wider community. Given these diverse influences, limitations, and pressures, the relationship between client and therapist and the knowledge the therapist brings to treatment can make the difference between success and failure. Drawing on her considerable experience and expertise, Kime provides readers with an understanding of these issues and the knowledge with which to assimilate and overcome their negative influences to achieve positive outcomes for the client and his or her family and immediate community.

Readers are provided with examples of different treatment programs for inpatients and outpatients including return to work, which is possible for a percentage of people with memory impairment who learn to compensate effectively. The heart of the book is, perhaps, the description of the compensations available and discussion as to how to teach clients to use them. Those engaged in memory rehabilitation know only too well that people who need memory compensations most urgently have the greatest difficulty in using them. This is because the act of using compensatory aids involves memory, the very attribute that needs rehabilitating. Teaching people with memory impairment how to use compensatory aids is where Kime's clinical experience and common sense shine through, and that is why this book will be essential reading for occupational therapists and psychologists who work in memory rehabilitation.

I remember observing Kime working with a young woman with dense amnesia when I was in Arizona. The woman was provided with a sophisticated date book (an organizer) that I considered to be too complicated for her. Undaunted, Kime taught the client to use this system very successfully through patience, ingenuity, and an intuitive awareness of such principles as implicit memory and errorless learning. Once she was able to compensate so effectively, doors were opened for the young woman, who was able to return to work, initially in a voluntary capacity and later as a paid employee.

—Barbara A. Wilson, PhD
Cognition and Brain Sciences Unit, Medical Research Council
Cambridge, England
Oliver Zangwill Centre for Neuropsychological Rehabilitation
Ely, England

Foreword

Susan Kime is an experienced occupational therapist who has been dedicated to helping clients with memory impairment learn to cope with those difficulties in day-to-day life. This book summarizes some of the basic facts that she has found helpful in teaching clients when compensating for memory deficits. The book, like its author, is practical and clinically useful.

This book centers around the practicalities of how to approach clients when teaching them memory compensation techniques. It also considers the variables that have to be considered to increase the probability that such training will be helpful. The book discusses important variables, such as characteristics of both client and therapist that may influence outcome. This type of analysis is frequently neglected in rehabilitation texts.

All of us are faced with a great deal of information that we need to process each day. With brain injury, this can be quite a confusing and frustrating task. By putting together some basic guidelines for teaching clients memory compensation techniques, Kime has contributed an important volume that will be helpful to occupational and speech and language therapists involved in brain injury rehabilitation.

—George Prigatano, PhD
Newsome Chair, Clinical Neuropsychology
Barrow Neurological Institute
Phoenix, Arizona

Introduction

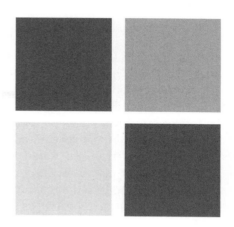

Background

I was 16 years old and living in a small midwestern town when I worked with my first "patient." I had never even heard of *occupational therapy*, but there I was working with a patient with mental retardation on work re-entry. At that time, the State of Minnesota was reintegrating patients who had been institutionalized into the community. The owners of a small "mom and pop" restaurant where I worked during the summer washing dishes had agreed to provide on-the-job training for one of those patients. I volunteered to teach her to wash dishes, figuring that it would make my job easier (like any teenager, I wanted all the free help I could get). And with the insight of a typical teenager, I did not realize that it would turn into a valuable learning experience, and eventually, a career.

Looking back over the past 30+ years and the hundreds of clients whom I have treated since my "first patient," I realize that the approach I had used with her included many of the fundamental aspects that make memory compensation training successful. Somehow, even though I was young and had no formal training, I managed to help her become gainfully employed.

I have spent my entire career working with clients with brain injury across all levels of rehabilitation, ranging from intensive care to outpatient programs. Many had memory problems, which is not surprising, as difficulty with memory is a common cognitive deficit experienced following injury to the brain (Freeman, Mittenberg, Dicowden, & Bat-Ami, 1992; Hutchison & Marquardt, 1997; Schacter, Rich, & Stamp, 1985). Over the years, I have worked with many therapists who have asked me for help when working with clients with brain injury to develop compensations for memory impair-

ment. Often the therapist does not know how to get started because the situation seems too complicated or overwhelming. Most of the time my advice is to start as simply as possible—try something reasonable, and see if it works. If it does not, try something else. That is what I did as a 16-year-old who did not know any better, and that is still the basis of my approach today.

I do not mean to suggest that it is easy. A lot of time and thought go into determining what is a practical and effective way to start with a new client. Therapists do not necessarily have to get everything right the first time. Even today I make lots of changes to treatment plans with clients as they progress. Part of this is just common sense; no two clients are identical in their deficits and needs, so how could the same approach work for everyone? Adjustments are almost always necessary. The key is to quickly recognize when things are not working and change them.

The Evidence and My Experience

I am often asked by fellow therapists about what is a "reasonable" way to start working with a new client with memory impairment. A first thing to assess is the level of awareness that the client has about his or her injuries and their effects on his or her daily life. Awareness is a complicated issue, and much has been written on this topic. For example, Flemming and Strong (1995) have described three levels of self-awareness after brain injury: (1) insight into injury-related deficits, (2) understanding of the impact of those deficits on everyday activities, and (3) a realization of how the deficits will affect future functioning. Similarly, Crosson et al. (1989) defined a self-awareness model with "intellectual awareness" at the base, "emergent awareness" at the middle, and "anticipatory awareness" as the highest level. In some instances, a client is completely unaware and may deny that he or she has any deficits at all (Prigatano & Klonoff, 1998).

It is generally accepted that clients who have a high degree of awareness of their problems are more likely to engage in the rehabilitation process. And the converse also is true. As stated by Prigatano (1992), "Patients cannot maintain a productive lifestyle unless they have come to face the realities of their life, and this means improving self-awareness and self-acceptance" (p. 60). At the same time, it is important to note that highly aware individuals are at greater risk for emotional distress (Fleming & Strong, 1995), so both overall awareness and emotional factors need to be considered.

I bring all of this up not just to prove that awareness is complicated but to point out that a primary factor that will help define an appropriate starting point for a new client is his or her level of awareness. As Fleming, Strong, and Ashton (1998) have stated,

> Deficits in self-awareness can seriously interfere with participation in rehabilitation by persons with TBI [traumatic brain injury], causing problems with motivation, engagement in therapy tasks, compliance with suggestions for behavioural change, and the use of compensatory strategies. (p. 39)

I would generalize this statement to include all injuries to the brain and not just TBI. My perspective on assessing a client's level of awareness and the impact that it has on determining appropriate treatment is included in Chapter 1.

This leads into my next point: simplicity. I do not mean to give the impression that only the most simple approaches are effective in developing memory compensations. But I do mean to say that when one begins working with a client, it is important to consider the level of complexity appropriate for that individual's situation. A personal example of the importance of starting simply relates to my favorite form of exercise—running. Not only does running provide me with a good physical workout, but I often do my best thinking while on a long run. Years ago when I first decided to try running, I started simple: I entered the walking portion of a local running event. I enjoyed it so much that the next time I signed up for the 5-K run. Since then I have run dozens of 10-Ks, half-marathons, and even a full marathon. If a trainer had approached me at my first running event with a comprehensive plan for running a marathon, I never would have signed up. But by starting simple and taking things at my own pace, I turned running into a way of life for me.

I believe that there are many parallels between my running experience and working with a client with memory impairment, not the least of which is that, as a therapist, one is trying to make use of memory compensations a way of life for the client. A necessary starting point is selection of an approach that is appropriate to the level of the individual. Ownsworth and McFarland (1999) reached this conclusion in a paper in which they stated, "remediation of memory impairment needs to be ecologically sound, by making procedures acceptable to patients in regard to their lifestyle, as well as appropriate to their level of cognitive deficits and stage of recovery" (pp. 619–620).

Relating this to awareness, if the client has little awareness of his or her deficits, then starting with a complex, multifaceted memory compensation system is almost certainly the wrong choice. The client probably will not even see the point in trying to use it. Furthermore, too much complexity at the beginning will lead to a frustrating situation where most of therapy time is spent trying to convince an uninterested client that he or she will benefit from the compensations. Ultimately this will make it more difficult to establish a good working relationship with the client, and establishing and maintaining a good working alliance are vital aspects of ensuring a successful treatment outcome (Prigatano et al., 1994). It is far more constructive to start with a simple approach and then build on its success to eventually arrive at an effective long-term memory compensation system that meets the psychological and lifestyle needs of the client. The approaches to accomplish this that have worked well for me are fully described in Chapters 2 and 3.

Another thing that I always consider when beginning to work with a new client is whether or not he or she would benefit from the use of an errorless-learning approach. The first time I heard the term *errorless learning* was in 1993 when Dr. Barbara Wilson visited the clinic where I was working. She had observed my treatment of a client with dense amnesia as we worked on memory compensations focused on the use of a day planner. Afterward, she commented that I had been using an "errorless-learning approach." I was not sure what she meant and asked for an explanation. Dr. Wilson indicated that I had been using a treatment approach which, by design, was eliminating errors from client's responses. She went on to say that my approach actively directed my client to the correct responses. This is, in essence, the definition of errorless learning. In a 1996 paper, Wilson explained the basis for errorless learning as follows:

Most of us can learn from or benefit from our errors because we remember our mistakes and, therefore, avoid making the same mistake repeatedly. People without episodic memory, however, cannot remember their mistakes, so [they] fail to correct them. Furthermore, the very fact of engaging in a behaviour may strengthen or reinforce that behaviour. Consequently, for someone with a severe memory impairment, it makes good sense to ensure that any behaviour which is going to be reinforced is correct rather than incorrect. (p. 53)

Baddeley and Wilson (1994) have demonstrated that this technique is particularly effective when working with clients with amnesia. Over the past decade, the errorless-learning approach has become widely accepted as a practical, effective technique to facilitate memory performance (Clare et al., 2000; Kerns & Thomson, 1998). I have found that nearly all of my clients benefit in one way or another from the use of errorless learning. Additional discussion of this is included in Chapter 3. Case studies including descriptions of how I have incorporated an errorless-learning approach into the treatment plans of several clients are provided in Chapter 4.

Another aspect of working with clients with memory impairment that I emphasize is the importance of observing and working with the client in his or her functional environment. I often find that new therapists have never even considered the idea that they should get out of the clinic and observe the client at work, home, or school to establish appropriate therapy goals and gauge the effectiveness of treatment. I summed it up this way in a paper I wrote with Dr. George Prigatano: "The importance of treating the patient at the home or work site cannot be overstated. It provided a clear picture of what compensations were, in fact, working well and which had to be modified" (Prigatano & Kime, 2003, p. 50). It also brings with it the opportunity to obtain feedback from the people closest to the client (e.g., family, friends, teachers, co-workers) and to train them to assist in the treatment plan (Burke, Danick, Bemis, & Durgin, 1994; Kerns & Thompson, 1998).

A further benefit of working with the client in his or her functional environment relates to awareness. The impact that "real-life" settings can have on a client's ability to recognize his or her memory deficits is demonstrated in a study published by Dirette in 2002, who reported working with a client who was

participating in several cooking tasks while in the cognitive rehabilitation programme. She did not, however, gain the awareness of her cognitive

deficits until she attempted to cook in her own kitchen. A client may be able to rationalize poor performance in the clinic or may not have the abstract reasoning needed to comprehend their cognitive deficits. (p. 868)

It also should be noted that awareness facilitated by a real-life setting can sometimes take years to develop. Wilson (1991) reported finding evidence of increased use of memory compensations by patients 5 to 10 years after they had experienced a brain injury. Wilson hypothesized that the reason that these patients did not immediately adopt the memory aids introduced to them during memory therapy "might have something to do with subjects themselves recognizing (possibly under the influence of relatives) the need for such aids as they were confronted by problems associated with the actuality of daily living" (p. 131). Wilson went on to state that "It follows that the use of aids would be more effectively taught in the environment in which they are to be used" (p. 133). Several examples of the work that I have done with my clients in their functional environments can be found throughout this book.

About This Book

So, with much already written about the benefits of using memory compensations with clients with brain injury, why did I feel it necessary to write this book? In one word, the answer is *implementation*. Although many researchers in this area have agreed on the benefits of memory compensation training (see, e.g., Carney et al., 1999; Cicerone et al., 2000), and research papers containing general guidelines for memory compensation strategies are common (see, e.g., Burke et al., 1994; Fleming, Shum, Strong, & Lightbody, 2005; Ownsworth & McFarland, 1999; Prigatano & Kime, 2003; Sohlberg, White, Evans, & Mateer, 1992; Zencius, Wesolowski, Krankowski, & Burke, 1991), to my knowledge nothing that provides detailed specific instructions for the implementation of external memory aids has been published. In 1997, Hutchinson and Marquardt observed that

Most rehabilitation clinicians receive little or no explicit training in treatment of memory impairments but frequently express a need for treatment methods appropriate to the brain-injured population and find themselves uncomfortably improvising or using memory-improvement routines designed for the non-brain-damaged population. (p. 51)

The following year, Donaghy and Williams (1998) went on to say,

In patients with severe disorders there is a relative lack of explicit and readily accessible protocols published in the literature that clinicians can use in their work. In the absence of such protocols, it is difficult for clinicians to know exactly how to proceed with the business of training this most difficult population of patients. (pp. 1061–1062)

This was the situation when I began working on this book, and now in 2006, as it is finally going to press, not much has changed. This lack of specific detailed guidelines might be explained by the fact that external memory aids are commonly used by all of us. We all use calendars, watches, and alarm clocks to help us keep track of time. Many of us also use personal organizers, filing systems, lists, and so forth to help us remember things. Although we may be able to get along without them, using calendars, to-do lists, checklists, and forms often helps us be more organized and efficient. Because these items are so common, it may seem reasonable to assume that a client with memory impairment would be familiar with them and have no difficulty using them.

My experience, however, has shown me that this is not the case. Over and over again I find that the most difficult part of memory compensation training is getting the tools fully integrated into the daily routines of the client. Kapur (1995) put it this way:

There is a fallacy that memory aids may simply be given to patients to use, and little intervention is required from the therapist. If only this were the case! . . . The patient needs to be trained to recognise situations where a memory aid of the appropriate kind will be of particular use and must develop motivation to set about using it effectively. (p. 546)

Successful treatment is not simply a matter of giving the client a recommendation such as "get yourself a personal organizer." In almost every case (in fact, I cannot think of a single case of mine in which this was not true), much time and hard work are required. In a case reported by Sohlberg and Mateer (1989), it took more than 6 months of intensive training for a client with severe impairment to learn to independently use a simple memory notebook. This is echoed in my own experience with a client with a similar impairment with whom I had worked intensively in a full-day treatment program for more than 4 months (Kime, Lamb, & Wilson, 1996).

Although memory compensation training often is labor intensive, the rewards to the client can be great. The value to the client, both emotional and financial, of increased independence will be realized for a lifetime. Several studies have shown that the degree to which a client is able to compensate for memory deficits often defines his or her capability to function at work, at home, and socially (Kime et al., 1996; Wilson, 1991). In recent years, there has been an increased emphasis in the literature on the value of memory compensation strategies in relation to quality-of-life issues for clients with impairments. As Hutchinson and Marquardt (1997) have observed, "Long after most physical disabilities have reached stabilization or recovery, lingering memory problems prevent many survivors of brain injury from returning to active employment, independent living, or full social lives" (pp. 45–46). For such clients, memory compensations are an important aspect of regaining at least some of their former quality of life. Evans, Wilson, Needham, and Brentnall (2003) have supported this, saying,

Among rehabilitation professionals, there is a broad consensus that the most effective way of helping such individuals [those left with permanent memory impairments following injury to the brain] to cope with everyday life is through the use of compensatory strategies. (p. 925)

My intention as I started the task of putting down on paper the techniques I use with my clients with memory impairment was to create a concise "how-to" manual. During the past few years as I worked on this project, my "manual" has grown much larger than I envisioned, but I have tried not to lose sight of my initial intention. What I have attempted to create here is a practical book outlining the elements of the systematic approach I use when working with clients to implement compensations for their memory impairment.

Memory disorders occur in people with a variety of diagnoses, such as TBI, stroke, aneurysm, brain tumor, epilepsy, Parkinson's disease, and multiple sclerosis. The approach in all of these cases is similar. The chapters in this manual follow the sequence that I use when starting with a new client. Chapter 1 discusses assessing the client's readiness to begin memory compensation training. Chapter 2 explains how to identify the client's needs and the appropriate types of tools and strategies to meet them. Chapter 3 gives a structured approach to implementing memory compensation strategies and assessing their effectiveness. Chapter 4 includes several case studies that illustrate the use of the techniques described in the previous chapters. The case studies I have chosen illustrate how this structured approach can work with a variety of clients in different phases of rehabilitation.

Epilogue

And what became of that "first patient" whom I described at the beginning of this introduction? She recently retired after a 30-year career as a food service worker in a small-town grade-school cafeteria. Because she had good family and community support, she was able to live by herself in a home of her own. She has been able to enjoy a quality of life that she never would have had living in an institution. To this day, her success continues to inspire me to help others achieve an increased level of independence and a better quality of life.

References

Baddeley, A., & Wilson, B. A. (1994). When implicit learning fails: Amnesia and the problem of error elimination. *Neuropsychologia, 32*(1), 53–68.

Burke, J. M., Danick, J. A., Bemis, B., & Durgin, C. J. (1994). A process approach to memory book training for neurological patients. *Brain Injury, 8,* 71–81.

Carney, N., Chestnut, R. M., Maynard, H., Mann, N. C., Patterson, P., & Helfand, M. (1999). Effect of cognitive rehabilitation on outcomes for persons with traumatic brain injury: A systematic review. *Journal of Head Trauma Rehabilitation, 14,* 277–307.

Cicerone, K. D., Dahlberg, C., Kalmar, K., Langenbahn, D. M., Malec, J. F., Bergquist, T. F., et al. (2000). Evidence-based cognitive rehabilitation: Recommendations for clinical practice. *Archives of Physical Medicine Rehabilitation, 81,* 1596–1615.

Clare, L., Wilson, B. A., Carter, G., Breen, K., Gosses, A., & Hodges, J. R. (2000). Intervening with everyday memory problems in dementia of Alzheimer type: An errorless learning approach. *Journal of Clinical and Experimental Neuropsychology, 22,* 132–146.

Crosson, B. C., Barco, P. P., Velozo, C. A., Bolesta, M. M., Werts, D., & Brobeck, T. (1989). Awareness and compensation in post-acute head injury rehabilitation. *Journal of Head Trauma Rehabilitation, 4,* 46–54.

Dirette, D. (2002). The development of awareness and the use of compensatory strategies for cognitive deficits. *Brain Injury, 16,* 861–871.

Donaghy, S., & Williams, W. (1998). A new protocol for training severely impaired patients in the usage of memory journals. *Brain Injury, 12,* 1061–1076.

Evans, J. J., Wilson, B. A., Needham, P., & Brentnall, S. (2003). Who makes good use of memory aids? Results of a survey of people with acquired brain injury. *Journal of the International Neuropsychological Society, 9,* 925–935.

Fleming, J. M., Shum, D., Strong, J., & Lightbody, S. (2005). Prospective memory rehabilitation for adults with traumatic brain injury: A compensatory training programme. *Brain Injury, 19,* 1–10.

Fleming, J. M., & Strong, J. (1995). Self-awareness of deficits following acquired brain injury: Considerations for rehabilitation. *British Journal of Occupational Therapy, 58,* 55–58.

Fleming, J. M., Strong, J., & Ashton, R. (1998). Cluster analysis of self-awareness levels in adults with traumatic brain injury and relationship to outcome. *Journal of Head Trauma Rehabilitation, 13*(5), 39–51.

Freeman, M. R., Mittenberg, W., Dicowden, M., & Bat-Ami, M. (1992). Executive and compensatory memory retraining in traumatic brain injury. *Brain Injury, 6,* 65–70.

Hutchinson, J., & Marquardt, T. P. (1997). Functional treatment approaches to memory impairment following brain injury. *Topics in Language Disorders, 18,* 45–57.

Kapur, N. (1995). Memory aids in the rehabilitation of memory disordered patients. In A. D. Baddeley, B. A. Wilson, & F. N. Watts (Eds.), *Handbook of memory disorders* (pp. 533–536). Chichester, England: Wiley.

Kerns, K. A., & Thomson, J. (1998). Case study: Implementation of a compensatory memory system in a school-age child with severe memory impairment. *Pediatric Rehabilitation, 2*(2), 77–87.

Kime, S. K., Lamb, D. G., & Wilson, B. A. (1996). Use of a comprehensive programme of external cueing to enhance procedural memory in a patient with dense amnesia. *Brain Injury, 10,* 17–25.

Ownsworth, T. L., & McFarland, K. (1999). Memory remediation in long-term acquired brain injury: Two approaches in diary training. *Brain Injury, 13,* 605–626.

Prigatano, G. P. (1992). Neuropsychological rehabilitation and the problem of altered self-awareness. In N. von Steinbuchel, D. Y. von Cramon, & E. Poppel (Eds.), *Neuropsychological rehabilitation* (pp. 55–65). New York: Springer-Verlag.

Prigatano, G. P., & Kime, S. K. (2003). What do brain dysfunctional patients report following memory compensation training? *NeuroRehabilitation, 18,* 47–55.

Prigatano, G. P., & Klonoff, P. S. (1998). A clinician's rating scale for evaluating impaired self-awareness and denial of disability after brain injury. *Clinical Neuropsychologist, 12,* 56–67.

Prigatano, G. P., Klonoff, P. S., O'Brien, K. P., Altman, I. M., Amin, K., Chiapello, D., et al. (1994). Productivity after neuropsychologically oriented milieu rehabilitation. *Journal of Head Trauma Rehabilitation, 9*(1), 91–102.

Schacter, D. L., Rich, S. A., & Stamp, M. S. (1985). Remediation of memory disorders: Experimental evaluation of the spaced-retrieval technique. *Journal of Clinical and Experimental Neuropsychology, 7,* 79–96.

Sohlberg, M. M., & Mateer, C. A. (1989). Training use of compensatory memory books: A three-stage behavioral approach. *Journal of Clinical and Experimental Neuropsychology, 11,* 871–891.

Sohlberg, M., White, O., Evans, E., & Mateer, C. (1992). Background and initial case studies into the effects of prospective memory training. *Brain Injury, 6,* 129–138.

Wilson, B. A. (1991). Long-term prognosis of patients with severe memory disorders. *Neuropsychological Rehabilitation, 1,* 117–134.

Wilson, B. A. (1996). Rehabilitation and management of memory problems. *Acta Neurologica Belgica, 96*(1), 51–54.

Zencius, A., Wesolowski, M. D., Krankowski, T., & Burke, W. H. (1991). Memory notebook training with traumatically brain-injured clients. *Brain Injury, 5,* 321–325.

Identifying the Needs of Clients With Memory Deficits and Understanding the Traits of a Successful Therapist

Many factors influence the degree to which a given client will benefit from memory compensation training. Foremost is the client's ability to recognize his or her own memory problems. Those clients who are unable to recognize or have limited insight into their problems usually will not participate in the treatment. Another major factor is family and workplace support. Clients spend the majority of their time outside therapy sessions and must learn to generalize the skills learned in therapy to fit their personal circumstances. This will be successful only if the client's support network perceives the value of the treatment and participates in the process. Equally important to the efforts of the client and his or her support network are the organizational skills and level of commitment of the therapist.

Client Traits

Awareness

The client must have some awareness of his or her problems for the treatment to be successful. Many clients do not admit their memory problems until confronted with clear, undeniable evidence. Often clients must forget something of vital importance to them before they will make a real attempt to participate in memory compensation training.

For example, I had a teenage client who had obvious and frequent memory failures but was unconvinced that they would have any effect on his life outside therapy. I had tried for weeks to get him to begin to use a personal organizer, but to no avail. That changed one Monday morning when he showed up at therapy anxious to begin using an organizer. I thought, "Finally I've broken through, and he's listening to me." However, it turned out that he had completely forgotten a Saturday night date with a girl he really liked. For this client, forgetting this date was what was needed to get him started.

Many times clients are partially aware of their problems but do not realize the full extent of them. They may believe that they forget things infrequently and have a slight memory problem when, in fact, it is quite severe. Usually these clients are willing to begin memory compensation training but believe they will use it on a limited basis, such as only for tracking appointments. This initial limited use is often the first step that a client takes toward realizing the extent of his or her problems. Once the client observes the usefulness of the system in one area, he or she may realize that it also can be of help in other areas. For example, a client who begins by recording only appointments may soon recognize the system's usefulness for prioritizing tasks or keeping personal notes.

Clients who are completely unaware of or who actively deny their deficits are usually unable to benefit from memory compensation training. Attempts to pressure these clients into participating in treatment are likely to be a frustrating waste of time for both the client and therapist. It is much better to allow the client to develop awareness at his or her own pace and then begin treatment when he or she is ready. In such cases I make it clear to the client and family that I am available should the client later decide that treatment would be helpful. I've had many clients who have returned for treatment months, or even years, after our initial contact.

I cannot emphasize enough how important it is to allow clients to come to therapy when *they* are ready, even when their memory problems are evident to everyone but themselves. I've witnessed many cases in which therapists demanded that such a client participate in therapy, but I've never witnessed a case in which that approach worked. The most common outcome is that the working alliance with the client is fractured, and he or she will not return for services even when he or she later becomes aware of his or her problems. It is much more productive to "plant the seed" of what is available to the client and allow it to take root on his or her own terms.

Emotional State

Closely tied to the client's awareness is his or her ability to accept and deal with his or her memory impairment. In my caseload clients often experience a sudden and catastrophic event, such as stroke or head injury, that creates profound changes in their lives and those of their families. The first order of business is to determine if the client is emotionally ready to engage in treatment.

Clients who have experienced a brain injury often exhibit depression, heightened anxiety or, less frequently, paranoia in reaction to their situation. The therapist must be able to gauge the severity of such emotions in relation to the client's ability to actively participate in therapy. Clients with severe depression or who are anxious or have paranoia are poor candidates for treatment because they are unable to devote the effort necessary to be successful. Because participation in memory compensation training often confronts the client with his or her memory failures, it may exacerbate such emotional problems. With such clients there is no point to proceeding until their emotional state is under control. In fact, attempts to proceed may actually be detrimental to the client. In such cases, psychological or pharmacological treatment must be pursued prior to memory compensation training. It is best to refer such clients to neuropsychologists and physiatrists who are trained to address such issues.

However, I've found that clients who are only mildly depressed or anxious are likely to appreciate the benefits of using memory compensations. In fact, if disorganization is contributing to the depression or anxiety, using memory compensations may itself help provide a structure that facilitates recovery. I've included an example of this in Chapter 4. It involves a former client who had mild depression and was anxious because of her inability to organize her day and care for her family. Once she began working with me on using specific techniques to complete her daily responsibilities, she received much positive feedback from her family and again saw herself as a contributing family member. This had a very positive effect in reducing her depression.

Personality Traits

We all have personality traits that influence the way we live our lives. Some people are more flexible in adapting to change than are others. Some are more organized or more independent. Certain people are very predictable, while others are impulsive. When setting goals with the client, the therapist must consider the effect that such personality traits will have on the success of the treatment.

Through experience I've learned that clients who were disorganized prior to their injury are more likely to lack the discipline necessary to follow a structured system. Clients who had good organizational skills prior to their injury have a higher probability of success. This seems like common sense, but I've learned it the hard way. Early in my career I worked very hard with certain clients to make them use a system that I felt would work well, without regard for their personality and personal goals. Despite my best efforts, this approach almost always ended in failure. Eventually I learned to take a serious look at the client's personality before defining the goals of treatment.

To assess how a new client's personality traits will influence the treatment, I generally ask him or her and his or her family a series of questions such as

- Did you consider yourself to be an organized person before your injury?
- How did you remember to get things done at work (and home)?
- Were you a list maker? Or did you rely mostly on your memory?
- Did you use a personal organizer (paper or electronic)?
- What kind of a system did you have for paying your bills and keeping track of other paperwork?

I have no absolute formula for determining how the client's personality will influence the treatment plan. However, the answers I get to questions like those above give me a sense of how to begin treatment. This is just one factor among many to consider, but it definitely should not be overlooked.

I once had a client who remembered to do things throughout the day by writing them down on pieces of paper and putting them in his pocket. Prior to his brain injury, this method worked fine for him. Several times a day he would go through the papers in his pocket to remind him of appointments, telephone calls to make, and other tasks. When he completed a task, he threw out the piece of paper.

After his brain injury he came to me because he was having difficulty remembering to do things. He explained his "paper-in-pocket" system and showed me how he used it. His system clearly was not working. All of his pockets were crammed with scraps of paper. None of them was dated. He could not tell me whether the tasks he had notes for were complete or not. We sorted through them and determined that many of them were very old and no longer relevant.

For several weeks I worked with him to begin using an alternate method to track information and ensure that it was completed on time. The entire time he was very resistant. He told me many times that his system used to work very well for him—he never had any problems with it. I repeatedly attempted to get him to try a different approach so that he could compare the benefits to his system. The more I pushed, the more strongly he pushed back, until he finally chose not to participate in therapy any more. His personality was such that he did not possess the flexibility required to consider using a different system.

If I were given the chance to start over with that client, I would approach things differently to account for his inflexibility. Rather than pushing him to adapt to a completely new system, I would attempt to work with him to improve his "paper-in-pocket" system. Rather than trying to get him to use a formal personal organizer, I would try finding him a very small spiral-bound notepad that would fit in his pocket. By using that instead of separate pieces of paper, his notes would at least be in chronological order. Maybe I would eventually have been able to get him to write the date on the pages. Once a task was completed he could have torn

out the page and thrown it away. Unfortunately I disregarded his personality and his inflexibility, and as a result I did not help him.

The assessment of client traits I've detailed above is summarized in Figure 1.1. If the client has difficulty in any of the areas of awareness, emotional state, or personality, he or she probably is not ready to begin memory compensation training. These issues must be addressed before proceeding. If, on the other hand, the client has adequate awareness of his or her problems, is emotionally stable, and is motivated to work, then he or she is a good candidate to begin treatment.

Support Network

Family

Just as the client must be aware of his or her problems to benefit from treatment, the family also must have a realistic view of the client's deficits. Family members frequently underestimate the degree of impairment experienced by their loved one. This often contributes to, especially in the early stages of treatment, a reluctance to support therapy activities. As treatment progresses, family members usually develop a deeper understanding of how the client's deficits, which initially seemed so small, have profoundly affected their lives. Just as the treatment requires the client to focus on his or her deficits to improve, it also provides a means by which family members can objectively view the situation. This heightened family awareness usually leads to more thorough support of therapy goals.

One of my former clients came to our first session alone. He described the problems he was having running

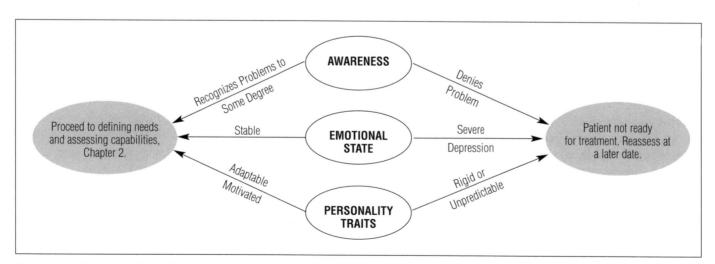

Figure 1.1. Assessment of client traits is needed to ensure that the client is ready to begin treatment.

his business. He felt that they were minor problems but nonetheless was frustrated by them. From his description I felt that he probably had more serious problems than he reported and that he would be unable to accomplish his normal job duties. I asked that he bring his wife to the next session to get her input.

Her assessment was that his memory impairment was having a greater impact than the client acknowledged, and she gave examples to support her view. However, despite recognizing more problems, she still felt that he was perfectly capable of running the business. But I suspected that the problems were more severe than either of them realized. Because she knew the business very well, and I would need her support for the treatment, I asked her to continue to attend all of the therapy sessions.

As the sessions progressed, both the client and his wife developed a deeper understanding of the significance of his impairments. His memory problems were having a much greater impact on his work activities than either of them had realized. Eventually she had to take a more active role in running the company, which was something neither she nor her husband had even considered before treatment.

I've seen many cases in which the client's memory impairment profoundly changes the dynamics of his or her family situation. Sometimes there is a role reversal that is resented by all parties. Consider a situation in which a dominant member of the family, for example, a male breadwinner, has a debilitating stroke. Suddenly he may find himself in a role where he is cared for by his family rather than providing for them. His wife may suddenly find herself in a role where she needs to lead the family and make decisions or perform tasks, such as paying the monthly bills, which she normally would have left to her husband. As a therapist it is important to recognize this type of situation and tailor therapy to address the immediate needs of not only the client but also the family.

I currently am working with a client whose situation very closely matches the above description. Before his injury his responsibilities included providing the income for the family as well as caring for their farm animals and upkeep of their property. His wife did not work outside the home but maintained the house and cared for their three children. He was referred to me 1 year after his TBI. He was physically capable of doing most of his former tasks at home, but memory problems prevented him from effectively completing them. He might feed one of the horses and forget about the others. A persistent complaint from his wife was that he would

begin to fill the watering trough and then forget to turn it off. She needed to follow up on all of his tasks to make sure they'd been done properly. She felt as if she had a fourth child to care for rather than a husband to help her. He was depressed and frustrated by his inability to complete what he considered simple tasks. This had gone on for a year and was close to destroying the family.

I knew from the start that I would be able to see this client infrequently—once every 2 weeks—because of the long distance from his rural home to my office. For the same reason it was not practical for me to provide treatment at his home. Therefore, the responsibility of providing the daily supervision he would need would have to fall on his already overwhelmed wife. There was no one else to do it. Somehow I needed to get his wife to the point where she could see the long-term benefits of her involvement in the treatment. Otherwise I wouldn't be able to help them.

During my initial evaluation it became clear to me that I needed to give them something concrete to help them right away. I couldn't tell them, "Come back in 2 weeks and I'll have something for you." We spent the majority of that first session making a list of tasks that this client needed to be able to complete independently. His wife helped prioritize the list. They left that day with a rudimentary, but functional, checklist that he could follow to make sure all of the animals were fed and watered. She committed to monitoring his use of the checklist each day to ensure that tasks were completed and then checked off the list.

From this small start we've continued to build an expanded checklist as well as other tools for him to use. As he gains independence with those tools, his wife no longer has to monitor his daily activities. He's becoming less frustrated as he's able to resume more and more of his pre-injury responsibilities. And his wife is not so overwhelmed. She attends and participates in every session I have with him. She has always been supportive, but as she sees the positive effects that using memory compensations is having, her resolve strengthens. Many issues remain, but their family situation is much less stressful. The progress we've made would have been impossible without his wife's support and active involvement.

However, not all families function well. Even when family members are fully aware of the client's deficits, they are sometimes unwilling or unable to participate in the treatment. In the worst cases, one or more of the family members may actively undermine the goals of the treatment. Although this is rare, it is important for the therapist to recognize it when it arises and take steps (possibly by referral to family counseling) to address this situation. Without the active support of the family, including help with defining the needs of the client, the client's potential for success is limited and therapy goals must be adjusted accordingly.

Recently I had a client who was referred to me following a severe stroke. She was a widow in her early 60s who owned and operated a very successful business. Her children also were involved in the business, but she was the leader. The stroke left her unable to perform any work duties. Her work was her life, so she was highly motivated to participate at some level, but she knew that she would not go back to leading the company.

I held a joint session with her and her son, who was now running the company, to define an approach to get her back to work. He had a realistic view of her deficits and was deeply saddened by the effect the stroke had had on his mother. We set up a work trial but soon determined that she would need constant supervision to complete anything worthwhile. Things were all right as long as I was there to provide that supervision, but company staff who I trained to work with her were frequently called away when I wasn't there. It soon became evident that the son did not feel that he could commit his own time or the company resources needed to allow his mother to return to work. Unfortunately, I had to discontinue therapy because no progress was being made. I can imagine a much different outcome had the family been able to provide more support.

One final point that needs to be made is that it is not fair for any therapist to insert his or her own family values into another family's situation. All families are different and capable of providing varying levels of support. As a therapist one needs to ask the family for their participation when needed, but it cannot be demanded. Therapy goals will need to be adjusted depending on their response.

Medical Staff

Inpatient treatment presents additional considerations. The client will interact with many staff members each day, which in some cases creates a chaotic environment. This is especially true for clients who are in a confused state, and the primary treatment emphasis is on basic orientation. To avoid potential problems, a consistent medical team that understands and follows treatment guidelines is required. This means that each of the client's providers must be aware of and supportive of the treatment plan. In situations in which consistency of care is not available, only limited goals are likely to be achieved, and the pace of progress will be slow.

I learned a lot about the importance of consistency early in my career while working on an inpatient rehabilitation unit. I was developing treatment plans that required the participation of the entire medical staff. Often I was working with clients on basic orientation components (e.g., person, place, time). I would solicit the help of all staff, from the custodian to the neurologist, who would come in contact with the client. I asked each of them to review the basic orientation information every time they saw the client. Sometimes I noticed substantial improvement in a given client on certain days and not on others. I soon realized that some members of the staff weren't participating, and I had no authority to force them. What I could do was to explain the benefits of their participation and ask for their cooperation. Gradually I learned who would participate and who wouldn't, and when I had a client who needed consistency I would try to arrange for him or her to be cared for by the staff members who would follow through.

In recent years I've worked in a hospital where specialized treatment teams are established that focus on clients who are agitated and aggressive. The teams consist of highly skilled therapists and nurses who are dedicated to working with these clients to modify their behavior. Consistency is the key to behavior modification, just like it is for memory compensation training. I know from my experience that using a consistent approach for clients with memory impairment is beneficial. I am aware of a few programs in which specialized teams similar to those used for behavior modification are applied to clients with memory impairment. But such practice is not widespread, and I believe it should be.

Community

For clients with a memory impairment whose primary goal is to return to work or school, the involvement of teachers, work supervisors, and co-workers is essential. A supportive community network that encourages the client's efforts, that is willing to accommodate the client's special needs, and that helps set goals and monitor progress is vital to the success of treatment. A key aspect to making that happen is good communication between the therapist and workplace or school. If communication is poor, the therapist and client will lack the necessary feedback to ensure continued improvement, and efforts to provide appropriate treatment will eventually fail.

I've worked with many therapists who feel that they can effectively get all clients back to work or school without ever going to the worksite. I could not disagree more with that approach. There are exceptions, but in nearly all cases it is essential to visit the workplace or classroom to observe how things are run and what the client's role is in that environment. A phone call to a supervisor or teacher is a good first step in opening communication channels but typically yields only a superficial amount of information compared to actually visiting the site and meeting him or her in person. The well-known saying "A picture is worth a thousand words" comes to mind. It may take weeks of phone calls and e-mails to get the same amount of information as a 1-hour visit. Many therapists I work with say they don't have the time to visit the client's worksites, but my feeling is that I don't have the time not to.

When I visit a worksite, I go there with two areas of focus in mind. First, I want to learn the details of the client's job. And second, I want to establish a good working relationship with the client's co-workers and management to foster good communication. Both are essential to having a successful outcome. Usually it doesn't take more than one or two visits before I'm able to gauge the extent of the commitment that management is willing to make and how much they'll be willing to adapt to the needs of the client. If they cannot be flexible and are unable to devote company resources to facilitating the client's transition back to work, then the progress will be slow at best. At worst, it may not be possible for the client to return to work.

There are rare instances in which it is not possible to go to the client's worksite. I once had a client who was a computer repair technician and traveled to a different job site every day. He had no central office. But even in that case I was able to arrange weekly meetings with him and his colleagues. His supervisor agreed to let me participate in their weekly breakfast meetings at a local restaurant. It wasn't a typical setting for a therapy session, but all of the right people were there each week, and it worked well. The client eventually returned to full-time work.

Constructive interaction with the support network is not only beneficial in understanding the extent of the client's problems and defining the goals of therapy but also is essential for monitoring progress. The only way I know to allow the client to reach his or her maximum potential for improvement is to enlist the help of the support network.

Therapist Traits

Most of the therapists I work with don't think of it this way, but I believe the therapist's role when working on memory compensation training with clients is similar to the role of a project manager. Many of the traits that the therapist needs are the same as those demonstrated by successful project managers in any business. The ability to communicate well, the willingness to assume a leadership role, strong organizational skills, and an objective and flexible approach to issues that inevitably arise are all essential elements. I work with some therapists who have excellent technical skills but who are not very good at working with clients with memory impairment because they don't possess project management traits.

Good Communication Skills

Most project management courses include a section on communication, because without good communication, a project will fail. The same is true when working with a client with memory deficits. Good communication among all segments of the client's support network (e.g., family, workplace, medical staff) is essential for effective treatment. The therapist must be willing to take the lead in facilitating this communication. As mentioned previously, each client spends only a small portion of his or her time in therapy sessions. The lessons learned in therapy are effective only if practiced throughout the day. A consistent approach that is followed by the entire support network is possible only if there is good communication.

Organized and Professional Treatment

Of course, fostering good communication is not enough by itself. Another key trait is the therapist's ability to demonstrate an organized, systematic approach to the treatment. If therapists are able to both communicate in words the effective use of memory compensation tools (such as a personal organizer) and demonstrate their use (by using a personal organizer themselves), then a client is more likely to learn. In essence, the therapist is modeling the behavior that he or she is trying to teach.

Frequently when I'm working with a client something will come up that I need to remember for the next session. Maybe I will need to bring an equipment catalog or a similar item to review with the client. Even if I probably won't need a reminder note, I use such situations as an opportunity to demonstrate to the client how I use the tools that I hope to teach him or her to use. I might say something like "I'd better write that down before I forget," then open my personal organizer (which I always keep with me) and show the client what I'm writing and where. In this way I've demonstrated the importance of always having the personal organizer available, immediately making entries when needed, where to make such entries, and how to write clear and concise notes.

In general, the client needs to see that the therapist is committed to the use of organizational tools. If the therapist is late for appointments and demonstrates poor follow-through on tasks, the client is unlikely to respect the therapist's ability to develop an effective treatment plan. Imagine what you'd be thinking if you attended a time management workshop that started 20 minutes late. Your confidence in the skills of the instructor would be greatly diminished. You might even get up and leave.

Being organized in your approach to members of the support network is important as well; otherwise, they too may lose confidence in your abilities. To get the full support of the client's family, co-workers, teachers, and so forth, they need to view you as a professional. Of course, being professional means different things to different people, but there are some qualities that most people will agree are necessary for one to be considered a professional. Being organized is one of them.

Whenever I have a client who is ready for a work trial, I arrange for a meeting with his or her supervisor. In many cases other employees at the company, such as a human resources representative, the department director, or a designated co-worker, also will attend the meeting. Such a meeting is a great opportunity to get the support of all the people needed to help with my client's transition back to work. They come to the meeting wondering what my plan is for the client and to what degree the company's resources will be needed. If I show up to the meeting without an agenda and with no recommendations for how to get started on the work trial, then I won't be able to establish the credibility needed to get their support. If, on the other hand, I am prepared to lead the meeting in an effective, organized manner, then I'll have a good chance of obtaining their cooperation. In many ways that first meeting is like an interview, and for it to go well I must make a good first impression. I want them to view me as a professional in the field of occupational therapy.

At such a meeting it is, of course, very important to arrive on time and wear business-like attire, just like you would for any job interview. In the hospital I normally wear casual clothing and tennis shoes because I spend part of each day with clients in the acute phase of their hospitalization. Before attending worksite meetings I change into clothing that is less casual—something more appropriate for a business meeting.

Boundary Setting

Another important therapist trait is the ability to set appropriate boundaries. Here, I'm referring to the emotional boundaries between a therapist and client. An aspect of professionalism is being objective. However, my experience is that many of the therapists I work with are very emotional and giving people. Maybe they were attracted to the health care field because of this aspect of their personality. Sometimes this emotional component overrides their objectivity.

More often than not, when working with clients with memory impairment, the situation is emotionally charged. Usually the client and his or her loved ones are just coming to grips with the change in their lives. As a therapist it is difficult to not become emotionally involved in the situation. The key is to maintain a healthy balance between an objective assessment of the situation and the sympathy you may feel. Sometimes this is the hardest part of being a good therapist.

During my career I've seen cases in which the therapist providing treatment becomes socially involved with the client and family. They may go to dinner together, exchange personal phone numbers, and visit each other's homes. Sometimes gifts are exchanged for birthdays and holidays. If the client has a family business, maybe goods or services will be exchanged for therapy. Although these things seem benign, they are a breach of the *Occupational Therapy Code of Ethics* (American Occupational Therapy Association, 2005) and are dangerous. They can lead to the destruction of the professional, therapeutic relationship that will most benefit the client. Imagine how difficult it would be to give unpleasant feedback to a client who you've become friends with. For example, what if the client becomes habitually late for therapy and because of your friendship you are unable to confront him or her about it? Or what if the client becomes dissatisfied with some aspect of your treatment but is unable to discuss it with you? It's easy to get into this kind of a mess without even realizing it. How does accepting an offer of theater tickets versus home-baked cookies from a client affect the therapeutic boundary? Each therapist may have a different opinion, but it is very important to consider your actions up front.

Learning From Mistakes

Because each client responds to treatment differently, failures in implementing treatment are inevitable. The therapist's ability to recognize the shortcomings of a treatment plan and adapt it to meet the client's needs is crucial.

One of my first clients when I began development of memory compensation strategies came to me with severe memory deficits caused by viral encephalitis. My first thought was that she would need a notebook that she could carry around with her to keep track of all of the information needed to manage her daily activities. I got her a 3-ring binder and divided it into multiple color-coded sections. Each section contained a different category of information. The color coding made cross-referencing very easy. To me it seemed like a great system. It seemed simple and straightforward.

I worked extensively with her on the use of the notebook for 2 weeks, but it resulted only in frustration and confusion. She was unable even to grasp the concept of the wonderful color-coded cross-referencing system I had developed. It was difficult for me to admit, but I'd devised a system that would work well for me (with my intact memory) but not for her. Eventually I realized that another approach was needed and simplified the approach. I began working with her on using a dry-erase board. Her family would simply write tasks, such as "feed the cat," that she needed to do that day on the board. I trained her to check the board often and erase tasks when completed. This was a big step down from the complicated notebook system I started with,

but it was the right first step for this client. With experience I've learned to quickly recognize situations in which my therapy approach is not working and make needed changes.

Summary

The successful treatment of a client with memory impairment starts with the client's awareness of his or her own problems and a desire to improve. A support network that understands and contributes to the goals of therapy is crucial. A therapist who is organized, professional, and adaptable to change completes the picture. When all of these pieces are in place, the greatest potential for a successful outcome is realized (see Figure 1.2).

Reference

American Occupational Therapy Association. (2005). Occupational therapy code of ethics. *American Journal of Occupational Therapy, 59,* 639–642.

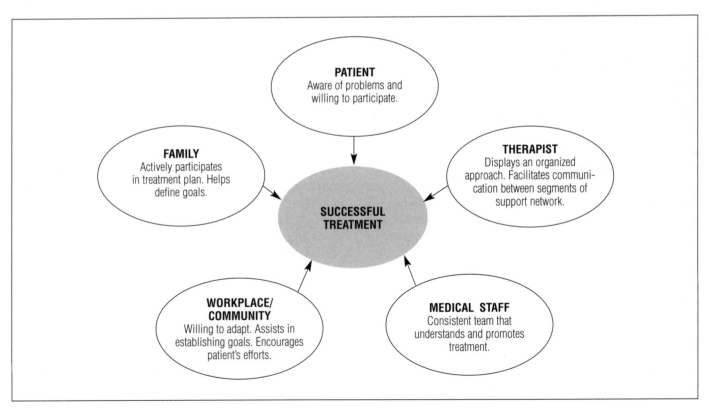

Figure 1.2. Successful treatment requires coordination of many efforts; any weak link jeopardizes the entire process.

Identifying the Best Compensatory System for Each Client

All candidates for memory compensation training arrive at therapy for the same reason: They need tools to help them meet their daily responsibilities. First and foremost, the therapist must determine what the client needs and desires to accomplish. It is usually necessary to observe the client outside the clinic (e.g., at home, work, school) to determine the goals of therapy. Such observation promotes interaction with those who have daily contact with the client and gives the therapist an opportunity to view the details of the client's life.

Once the client's needs are determined, the next step is to realistically assess the client's ability to use a system that meets those needs. What the client needs to accomplish and what can actually be done may not be the same. Cognitive, physical, and other deficits often prevent the client from fully using a compensatory system. The chosen system must be tailored to address such limitations.

In this chapter I define the memory compensation tools that I commonly use with my clients and then describe how to select and tailor a system that will meet the unique needs of an individual client.

Personal Organizers

My definition of a personal organizer is a structured, concise, portable tool that a person can use to track daily activities. People use personal organizers in the forms of calendars, day planners, notebooks, and electronic personal digital assistants (PDAs). A personal organizer should be structured and concise so that the information in it is easily accessible and quick to find. Being concise also allows it to be portable; if it is not portable, then it will not be readily available to enter and retrieve information when needed.

Virtually all commercially available personal organizers include a calendar (monthly, weekly, daily) and a telephone and address section. Some also include additional sections designed to meet specific needs, such as tracking finances. However, personal organizers currently available on the market are designed for use by the general public and almost always require customization to be useful for meeting the needs of a client with memory impairment.

Month-in-a-View Planning Calendar

Most people who are familiar with personal organizers have seen month-in-a-view calendars. In a paper (not electronic) organizer they generally span 2 pages, so that when the organizer is opened flat a full calendar month is shown (see Figure 2.1). This format offers very little space for writing notes. Usually, pages for each month of an entire year are included in this section of the organizer.

The client will use these pages to plan and track activities on a long-term basis, such as family gatherings, infrequent household chores, and monthly bill paying. This section is a good place to highlight important dates such as birthdays and anniversaries and also provides a long-term chronology of events that is useful for reference. It also provides a location for recording information that will later be transferred to daily pages, as it is sometimes impractical to carry an entire year's worth of daily pages in the organizer.

Daily or Weekly Dated Pages

In this section of a personal organizer the pages are arranged so that a single day or week is visible (see Figures 2.2A and 2.2B). Whether a client should use daily or weekly pages will depend on the amount of information to be recorded. Daily pages provide more space for note-taking than do weekly pages.

SUN	MON	TUES	WED	THURS	FRI	SAT
	JUNE S M T W T F S 1 2 3 4 5 6 7 8 9 10 11 12 13 14 15 16 17 18 19 20 21 22 23 24 25 26 27 28 29 30	AUGUST S M T W T F S 1 2 3 4 5 6 7 8 9 10 11 12 13 14 15 16 17 18 19 20 21 22 23 24 25 26 27 28 29 30 31			1 CANADA DAY (CANADA)	2
3	4 INDEPENDENCE DAY	5	6	7	8	9
10	11	12	13	14	15	16
17	18	19	20	21	22	23
24	25	26	27	28	29	30
31						

JULY 2005

Figure 2.1. Example month-in-a-view calendar.

Having pages that are preprinted with both the day and date can help avoid the confusion associated with including improperly dated pages in the organizer. I learned about the importance of this years ago when I asked a client to purchase pages for his personal organizer. He arrived at my next session with undated daily pages that required him to fill in the day and date by hand. He had taken the time to do this, but unfortunately he had made a mistake such that the day of the week did not properly match the date. Once we realized the mistake, we had to spend most of that session correcting it, because we couldn't proceed with learning how to use the organizer until the corrections were made. Valuable therapy time was wasted, and the client was embarrassed. Since then I have emphasized to clients and their families to purchase only pre-dated pages.

To-Do Lists

Tasks such as writing a letter to a friend or cleaning out the refrigerator, which need to be remembered but do not have to be completed on a particular day or at a specific hour, should be included in the personal organizer in "to-do" lists (see Figure 2.3). To-do lists provide a medium-to-long-range planning tool for activities. Once a specific time that an item will be accomplished is determined, it should be transferred from the to-do list to the daily pages. For example, if the to-do list contains a note to schedule a medical appointment, once the appointment is scheduled, the date and time of the appointment should be recorded in the daily pages.

I have had several clients who started treatment with an extensive to-do list but no means of organizing

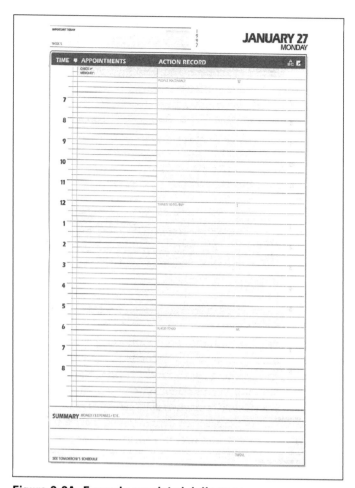

Figure 2.2A. Example pre-dated daily page.

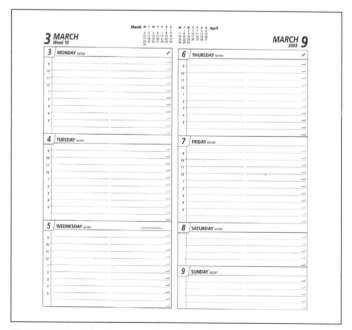

Figure 2.2B. Example pre-dated weekly page.

	TO-DO LIST	
Date	**Task**	**Date Completed**
3/2	Clean baseboards in hallway	
3/2	Clean out hall closet	3/5
3/5	Call charity to pick up old clothes	
3/10	Fertilize grapefruit tree	3/20
3/15	Drop off old books at VNSA	
3/20	Wash outside windows	3/27
3/27	Change oil in car	

Figure 2.3. Example to-do list.

it. They might have lists of tasks in many different places with no means of prioritizing them or documenting their completion. A recent client reported being "stressed-out" because she had sticky notes everywhere in her house and referred to herself as the "Queen of Post-It." Whenever she thought of something she needed to do, she would write it on a sticky note and affix it to the nearest surface, such as the kitchen refrigerator or a mirror in the bathroom. She quickly lost track of where all of her notes were. The first thing we worked on in therapy was to consolidate all of her notes into a single to-do list. Once we got all of her tasks recorded on one prioritized list, her anxiety greatly decreased.

Journal Section

This is a private section of the organizer reserved for clients to use at their discretion. Not all clients choose to use a journal section; it is most frequently used by clients with severe impairment as a kind of substitute long-term memory. It provides a location for these clients to record their innermost thoughts and feelings or anything else they might view as important and can play a significant role in providing a sense of continuity for the individual. No rules need to be followed for the formatting of this section, which usually consists of blank pages that the client can personally date if he or she so wishes. Because this is often an intensely personal section, the role of the therapist should be limited to offering the journal section as an option; it is not recommended for the therapist to ever review a client's private journal. However, journal entries often provide a basis for discussion if the client is participating in psychotherapy.

Electronic Organizers

Some of my clients, especially those who are interested in technology, are very interested in using an electronic organizer or PDA instead of the traditional paper organizer. At first glance, electronic organizers seem to have many benefits: They are small and portable; they can hold much information; and they may have clocks, alarms, or pagers built in. However, they have several critical weaknesses. First of all, it's not easy to enter and retrieve information, especially for clients with memory impairment. Because portable electronic organizers are too small to include a standard keyboard, notes are entered using a small keyboard or stylus, which is a challenge for most clients and can take a lot of time. Second, their small size is great for portability but also makes them difficult to read and easy to misplace. Finally, electronic organizers usually include lots of features that the client does not need. These extra features generally mean that there are extra menu items and operational modes that cause confusion. For these reasons, even without considering their added cost compared to paper organizers, I do not recommend electronic organizers for my clients at this time. I'm hopeful that in the near future a simple and easy-to-use electronic organizer that can meet the needs of some clients will be available on the market.

I've had several clients who insisted on using electronic organizers. One was a woman who had used a Palm Pilot for many years before her brain injury. She had one of the earliest versions with only limited features. She was very comfortable and proficient using it even after her injury. However, new learning was challenging for her because of moderate cognitive deficits, and I suspect that she would have difficulty learning to use any electronic organizer other than her trusty old Palm Pilot.

Another client who comes to mind was a computer technician who, when I first saw him, was learning to use an electronic organizer. His doctor used the same model and had recommended it to him. Being in a technical field, he was very excited about using it. After 2 weeks of working with him on the use of his new organizer, it became clear that it was too complicated for him. It took too long for him to enter notes, and he had difficulty paging through the menus to retrieve information. He didn't have any problem understanding how to use the organizer, but using it just took too much time. I eventually convinced him to try a paper organizer, which ended up working very well for him.

Forms, Checklists, and Procedures

Forms are customized pages designed to provide a record of activities related to a specific topic. Forms supply a means for clients to consolidate information on a subject so they can quickly refer to it later. The example in Figure 2.4 shows a common type of form consisting of a table that is filled in as the client completes activities. Many clients with memory impairment benefit greatly from using forms to keep track of what they have done.

Whereas forms provide a structured format for recording yet-to-be defined details of future activities, checklists provide a means of ensuring consistent performance of repeated activities that are already fully defined. In some cases the checklist specifies the sequence to be followed while carrying out a procedure and could be called a procedural checklist. In other cases, it simply enumerates tasks to be completed in no

HOMEWORK ASSIGNMENTS				
Date Assigned	Class	Assignment	Date Due	Handed In
11/9	Science	Read Pages 10–15. Complete problems 1–5 on page 16.	11/11	–
11/9	Civics	Write 100-word essay. See handout in Civics notebook.	11/20	
11/10	Math	Problems 5–15, page 89.	11/12	–
11/10	English	Term paper. See syllabus in English notebook.	12/15	
11/12	Science	Complete problems 4–11, page 52.	11/16	–
11/12	Math	Review pages 90–95. Do problems on page 95.	11/16	–
11/13	English	Book report. See outline in English notebook.	11/18	
11/16	Civics	Read pages 70–80. Answer questions 1–20 on page 80.	11/18	

Figure 2.4. Example form for tracking homework assignments.

particular order. The checklist shown in Figure 2.5 provides examples of both. The upper section (labeled "Appointment Needs") is simply a list of items to be gathered and brought to an appointment. The items don't have to be gathered in any particular order. The lower section (labeled "Client Meeting") lists in order the tasks to be completed during and after each client meeting. The sequence in which the tasks are completed is important; thus it is a procedural checklist.

Checklists are routinely used in many work environments to ensure accuracy and consistency in the performance of duties. An airline pilot using a checklist before takeoff is a good example. However, with clients with memory impairment, even a basic routine, such as taking medication, may require the use of a checklist. Checklists also can provide important documentation to verify what the client has actually completed, for instance, the taking of medication.

By providing a structured outline, checklists also help ensure that activities are completed correctly each time. For some clients the successful completion of activities on a checklist becomes routine, and they can eventually complete the activities without referring to the checklist. In this way the checklist is a very valuable tool for increasing the independence of some clients.

Because each client has unique needs regarding, for instance, his or her job functions at work or assignments at school, substantial time may be spent by the therapist assisting the client in creating the individualized forms and checklists. For some clients it is appropriate to include forms and checklists in separate sections of their personal organizer. Each section should have an individual tab to indicate its contents and allow the client to access it quickly.

Wristwatch With Hourly Chime

The most vital element for effective use of a memory compensation tool, be it a personal organizer, form, checklist, or procedure, is remembering to refer to it. This is particularly important for clients with memory impairment who may not fully understand the purpose of these tools or who may even forget that they have them. A digital wristwatch with an hourly chime and alarm is an inexpensive, commonly used, portable tool that provides a reliable means of prompting clients to use their compensation system.

For most people, wearing a watch is habitual. Even some of my clients with the most severe impairments still remember to put on a watch in the morning. Unlike a pager, phone, or other electronic device, the client is unlikely to leave the watch somewhere during the day.

WRITING A LIFE INSURANCE POLICY

Client: _____

Date: _____

Appointment Needs:

☐ Application form

☐ HIV consent form

☐ Life insurance buyer's guide and receipt

☐ Client file

☐ Policy illustration or non-illustration form

☐ Signature page

☐ Policy transfer form

Client Meeting:

☐ Confirm policy type with client

☐ Show policy illustration or sign non-illustration form

☐ Sign signature page

☐ Fill out application

☐ Sign HIV consent form

☐ Sign policy transfer form if applicable

☐ Obtain premium check and/or voided check

☐ Give buyer's guide and sign receipt

☐ Send application to insurance company

Figure 2.5. Example checklist.

A watch does not have to be removed to consult it and thus is less likely to be misplaced.

Many types of watches are available with features that range from simple to complex. The most basic digital watches have at least one alarm, but they don't always have an hourly chime. The most complex watches include appointment calendars and address books and can be linked to a computer for data transfer. My advice is, the simpler, the better. Most clients need only a basic watch that shows the time, day of the week, month, and date, with at least one alarm and an hourly chime. The more complicated the watch, the more likely it is that the client will have difficulty using it to reliably prompt him or her to use his or her memory compensation tool.

Other Memory Compensation Tools

Most of my clients benefit from using other basic memory compensation devices in conjunction with the tools described earlier.

Pillboxes

Nearly all of my clients take daily medications, and I always recommend that they use a pillbox to help organize them. Pillboxes are available with a wide range of features. The most basic have only a single compartment for each day of the week; deluxe models are available with timed-alarm dispensing systems that can be programmed for 7 days with multiple dosing times each day. Most of the time, I recommend a basic pillbox and attempt to add it to the client's daily routine.

Recently I had a client who needed to take medication with her morning meal and then again at bedtime. When I first saw her she reported difficulty remembering to take her pills at bedtime. She said that she was using a pillbox but that it was not working for her. It turned out that she kept her pillbox next to the coffeemaker in her kitchen. That strategy worked well for her morning pills because she always made coffee first thing in the morning. However, she was nowhere near the coffeemaker at bedtime. The solution was simple: I advised her to get another pillbox to keep on her nightstand. This fit perfectly into her existing daily routine: She would see one pillbox in the morning and the other at night. After that she had no problems remembering to take her medications.

It is common for anyone who is taking medications to at some time wonder whether or not he or she took the most recent dose. I suspect this has happened to all of us. In my experience with clients with memory impairment, I have seen that this is not just a once-in-a-while occurrence. It may happen daily, or even several times a day, and can cause much confusion and frustration for both the client and family. Pillboxes are great for confirming whether medication has or has not been taken. The pills are either still in the compartment, or they are not because they have been taken.

Another benefit of using pillboxes is that they provide an advance reminder to refill prescriptions that are running low. A pillbox is typically filled up for an entire week at a time. The process of filling the pillbox provides at least a few days of advance notice before a particular medication is depleted.

Timers

Timers are an inexpensive and easy-to-use tool that I frequently recommend for my clients. Timers are everywhere. Almost every home has at least one timer in the kitchen; in most cases there is one built into the range. I have never seen a digital watch that did not include a timer.

I teach my clients to use timers for tasks that they may forget to complete at a specific time, such as running a hose to deep water a tree. Using timers is very straightforward and does not require much explanation. Obviously a timer serves its purpose only if it is heard. For this reason I recommend portable timers that clients can keep with them. If the client is not using a watch, then I recommend using a timer that is small enough to fit into a pocket.

Many specialty timers are available for things such as turning on or off lights and appliances. One type I frequently recommend, and also use myself, fits on a garden hose and will turn off the water after a designated time. This is great for watering a tree or adding water to a swimming pool.

Electronic Spelling Checkers

Many of my clients have difficulty remembering how to spell words correctly. Depending on their situation this may not be a problem; however, I am currently working with several clients who are returning to work. Frequently misspelling words in e-mail or other written documents frustrates them and lowers the quality of their written communications. Most software used for business communication includes built-in spell checking, which helps with this, but it works well only if the misspelled word closely resembles the intended word. For instance, if the client phonetically spells the word *took* as *toch,* the online spell checker is unlikely to suggest the correct spelling. I've had clients who have spent 10 to 15 frustrating minutes trying to figure out the correct spelling in a case like this. The last thing they wanted to do was go through the embarrassment of asking someone else in their office for help.

Several clients with this type of problem have benefited greatly from the use of portable electronic spell checkers, which most office supply stores carry. Features include phonetic spell correction, definitions, synonyms and antonyms, and read-back capability (pronunciation of the word). Many are $20 or less. More expensive models also include games, calculators, and databanks for phone numbers and addresses. My advice is to select a model with only the features you think the client needs; features beyond what is absolutely needed usually make the spell checker confusing and difficult for the client to use.

Dry-Erase Boards

I tend to use dry-erase boards with my clients with more severe impairments who are not ready for a comprehensive personal organizer. A dry-erase board should be mounted in a prominent place where the client will encounter it frequently. This way he or she will be reminded of the items on it many times throughout the day. It is very important not to display too much information on a dry-erase board; otherwise, it will become cluttered and confusing to the client. I generally write on the board only basic orientation information (place and date) and possibly a simple activities of daily living (ADL) checklist that the client follows each day.

Daily maintenance of the dry-erase board is essential. Two common problems that interfere with the board's effectiveness are the failure to update the information and putting too many items on it. The hospital where I used to work had dry-erase boards in most patient rooms that showed the hospital name and the date. Of course, the date should have been updated early each morning, but that did not always happen. Often when I would enter a client's room and ask him or her to tell me the date, he or she would repeat the date written on the board, even if it was wrong.

It is important that someone (e.g., therapist, family member, medical staff) be designated to maintain the board daily. In the hospital, dry-erase boards attract many items. Visitors see them as a great place to write messages, show off their drawing skills, and tape up photos and cards. The board can quickly become very cluttered and difficult to read. If I ask for the date, the client may look at the board and not be able to clearly see the date or may be distracted by something on the board and forget what I asked. The person designated to maintain the board should clear off items that do not belong there and ensure that up-to-date information is always displayed.

Placards

Placards are simply signs that indicate when an activity is taking place. I often use them with my clients who are working on independence at home and are having difficulty completing routine tasks. A common problem is forgetting to promptly remove laundry from the washing machine. After several days the client may happen upon a damp, moldy pile of clothes in the washer. A solution that works well is a placard reading "Laundry in Progress" that is posted in a prominent place. Once the laundry is washed, dried, and put away, the placard is taken down. I usually have the client store the placard on top of the washing machine so he or she will have it available when he or she next does laundry.

There are many instances besides laundry for which a placard is an effective reminder. Sometimes I will use one instead of, or in conjunction with, a timer so that a client doesn't forget something. One of my former clients was easily distracted. Her family told me of several times that, when she would start to cook something and then get a call from a neighbor to come over for coffee, she would leave the house with the item simmering on the stove and maybe not come back for hours. The timer she had set on the stove would go off, but she would be away and never hear it. We were all worried that she would eventually start a house fire. I worked with her on using a placard that she would post on the exit door to her house before starting to cook. The placard said "Cooking—Don't Leave the House." Eventually she progressed to the point where she did not need the placard anymore and, thankfully, her house is still standing.

Designated Places

The final tool I want to discuss is really a strategy. I had a client who each morning would get into an argument with his wife and kids because he felt they had misplaced his wallet and car keys. Each day started badly, and the entire family was frustrated. I asked him where he would put these items each evening. Sometimes he would leave them in the kitchen, other times in the dining room or bedroom. He had no designated place for them.

The solution was straightforward. I suggested that he stop at a store on his way home from therapy and purchase a red plastic bin large enough for his wallet and keys. He placed the bin on the kitchen counter near the door so that he would pass by it each evening when he came home and each morning when he would leave.

Designated places are important for all clients with memory impairment because they cannot rely on their memory to backtrack and determine where they may have left something. Using a designated place is a simple strategy, but it is a strategy that is often overlooked.

Selecting the Proper Tools to Use With a Client

Interviews with the client and family usually yield several tasks that the client is having difficulty accomplishing. It may be that the client is still in the acute recovery phase and unable to complete even the most basic ADL. In other cases the client may have only mild impairments but is unable to perform job responsibilities at the same level that he or she could before the brain injury. Obviously the approach for setting up a personal organizer system would not be the same in each of these situations because the information that needs to be tracked, as well as the ability of the client to use memory compensation tools, is substantially different.

There are several factors to consider when selecting the memory compensation tools to use with a particular client.

Needs of the Client

One of the first things I ask new clients is, "What are you having difficulty doing?" I also usually ask a family member or someone who is with the client often what he or she has observed. On the basis of the answers I begin to understand the type of information that the client will need to track. If the client reports difficulty keeping track of the day and date, I know that we will start with a very limited system—maybe only a dry-erase board or a simple notebook. If, on the other hand, the client is back at work and wants to be a top performer, then more complex tools, such as detailed checklists and procedures, are likely to be needed.

I usually find that there are more issues than initially reported. Detailed questions and interviews with more than just the client are necessary. For example, clients who are focused on work may overlook home-related problems. In fact, I have never had a case in which a client who came to me for work-related problems did not have any issues at home. I often discover the home-related issues, such as an inability to pay bills on time, by questioning family members. Such issues could be the last thing on the client's mind.

Acuity of Injury

The acuity of the client's injury and the prognosis for recovery must be considered. Acute clients who have difficulty remembering such things as the therapy schedule, the day of the week, or why they are in the hospital may rapidly improve. For this reason, setting up an extensive memory compensation system to track such information may be pointless. The client may show substantial improvement quickly, even before he or she learns to use the tools. If it is important for an acute client to track such details, a simple notebook or dry-erase board may be all that is required.

If, on the other hand, the client is no longer in a rapid recovery phase and still has difficulty with basic information, an extensive system may be appropriate. The fundamental concept is to allow the client the time necessary to complete the initial phases of recovery before defining a comprehensive memory compensation system. Otherwise, time will likely be wasted by the therapist developing a system that will be inappropriate for the client in the long term.

Severity of Memory Problem

Assessment of the severity of the client's memory problem is critical in defining an appropriate memory compensation system. For example, clients with dense amnestic syndromes tend to require comprehensive compensation systems that provide a minutely detailed structure to their daily activities. This type of client typically is unable to learn new things and usually is unaware of his or her memory failures. On the other hand, clients with mild memory deficits may require a system with only a minimal level of detail. I like to think of it this way: "The bigger the memory problem, the bigger the organizer."

To assess the severity of a client's memory problem, it is helpful to review standardized memory test results, such as the Rivermead Behavioural Memory Test (Wilson et al., 1989) or the Wechsler Memory Scale (Reid & Kelly, 1993). However, such tests do not always identify functional memory loss. A client may show only mild impairment on a standardized test yet experience profound difficulty in meeting daily responsibilities. Standardized tests are administered in a sterile environment where distractions are minimized, which generally does not replicate the work or home environment of the client. Real-life distractions may severely impede the client's ability to remember. Although standardized tests do serve an important role, they are not a substitute for observing the client performing ADLs.

Cognitive or Language Deficits

To select an appropriate memory compensation system, it is necessary to understand the unique combination of cognitive or language impairments experienced by the client. If the client is unable to independently formulate coherent thoughts, verbally relate those thoughts, and physically write them down, he or she will have only a limited ability to use compensation tools. As mentioned earlier, clients who are not aware of their memory problems are often inappropriate for treatment. Clients with very severe cognitive deficits may lack the cognitive skills necessary to use memory compensation tools.

In most cases, however, the client's cognitive deficits are an obstacle that affect treatment goals but do not prevent treatment. The goals for clients with severe cognitive impairments are usually quite limited. Accordingly, the memory compensation system needed to reach these goals is usually quite basic. However, if the client's cognitive deficits are minimal, then more advanced treatment goals are likely to be achieved and a more comprehensive system to enable those goals is appropriate.

Physical Impairments

The therapist must select a memory compensation system that realistically addresses the client's physical limitations. If the client has difficulty writing, a system that does not rely heavily on the client's writing skills must be developed. For example, clients with ataxia are usually unable to write within the confines of a small space and require larger personal organizers. If a client's writing abilities are limited to simply checking a box, then a system that exclusively uses checklists or relies heavily on the use of customized rubber stamps may be appropriate.

It also is important to remember that for a compensation system to be effective, it needs to be with the client throughout the entire day. If the client has difficulty carrying a large personal organizer, then the use of a backpack, pouch on a wheelchair, or other adaptive measure should be considered.

Support Network

To begin a treatment plan, the therapist must understand the client's living or vocational environment. The client may be in a hospital or extended-care facility where many different staff members are involved in care. Or the client may be at home, where only a few family members provide care. In either case, for the

treatment to be successful, consistency is required. This means that each of the client's providers must be aware and supportive of the treatment plan.

In situations in which consistency of care is not available, only limited goals are likely to be achieved. The memory compensation system to reach those goals will be minimal. If a strong support network is available, more extensive goals and systems are appropriate.

Summary

The influence of the above-mentioned factors on the selection of a memory compensation system is diagrammed in Figure 2.6. Across the bottom of the figure are memory compensation systems ranging from the most to the least comprehensive. Separate consideration of each factor leads toward one or the other extreme. The combined effect of all factors usually leads to a system somewhere between the extremes. No attempt to provide a relative importance of the factors influencing the selection is made here. It is left to the judgment of the therapist to gauge the effects of each of these factors on the client's individual situation and to determine the appropriate memory compensation tools to use.

A former client of mine provides an example that illustrates the consideration of all of the previously mentioned factors when defining an appropriate memory compensation system. She lived in an apartment with her mother, who had a physical disability. For years my

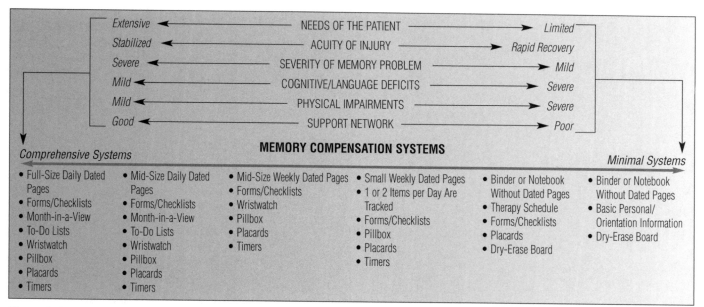

Figure 2.6. Detailed evaluation of client capabilities in many areas is necessary to define an appropriate system.

client had had a seizure disorder, and one day she had a seizure while crossing a street. She was hit by a car and sustained a brain injury.

Before her accident she was able to do limited volunteer work, but afterward this was no longer possible. When I saw her it was more than a year after the injury and was well past any rapid recovery phase. She had only mild cognitive and language and physical impairments but severe memory deficits. Because of her poor memory, she needed to track extensive amounts of information. She could not remember things from day to day; for instance, she would repeatedly rent the same movies from the local video store. She could not remember to keep appointments, make phone calls, or take her medications.

All of these factors indicated the need for a comprehensive memory compensation system. However, the client did not have a strong support network. Her mother was unable to participate in any therapy sessions and, because of her own physical problems, could not provide any assistance for the client at home. There were no friends or other family members who could assist. This single factor greatly limited the therapy goals. I knew the client could benefit from a personal organization system, including personalized forms, checklists, and a wristwatch with an hourly chime or alarm. However, I also knew that she would need a strong support network to learn to use such a system. My working with her in therapy sessions for only a few hours each week would not be enough. She would need someone to constantly prompt her to use the system throughout the day and to provide feedback concerning things that were not working that therefore needed modification. In the end, we defined a minimal system that was limited to a pillbox and a small notebook with only one customized form that she used for keeping track of appointments, paying monthly bills, and managing her daily medications.

This example illustrates how important it is to review each factor and gauge its influence on the selection of memory compensation tools. Rarely, if ever, is it a "black-and-white" decision. The sound judgment of the therapist is necessary to define an appropriate system.

References

Reid, D. B., & Kelly, M. P. (1993). Wechsler Memory Scale: Revised in closed head injury. *Journal of Clinical Psychology, 49,* 245–254.

Wilson, B., Cockburn, J., Baddeley, A., Hiorns, R., Smith, P., Ivani-Chalian, R., et al. (1989). *Rivermead Behavioural Memory Test* (RMBT). Titchfield, UK: Thames Valley Test Company.

Implementing Memory Compensation Strategies and Assessing Their Effectiveness

Once the needs of the client are defined and the appropriate memory compensation tools are identified, then the hard work of teaching the client to use the chosen system begins. Because each client has a unique combination of needs and abilities, there is no standard formula for implementation. A customized approach is always needed. Even the most experienced therapist will probably have to modify the approach many times during the treatment of a given client. The therapist's ability to learn from initial failures and make necessary modifications to the treatment plan is an essential element of the process.

Implementation Cycle

Development of an effective memory compensation system is a learning process that requires frequent review and modification as it evolves toward success. A repeated cycle of learning that consists of (1) planning and establishing goals, (2) executing the plan to meet those goals, (3) measuring the degree of success, and (4) modifying the treatment approach to achieve greater success is necessary.

The sections that follow provide guidelines for the therapist to follow while working through the four phases of the implementation cycle (see Figure 3.1). For clarity, these phases are described as distinct segments. However, they do not necessarily occur in a well-defined sequential order. As this approach is used, it will become clear that the phases usually overlap. For instance, it is common that the measurements of the treatment's success are made as the client uses the system (execution phase) and modifications are made whenever necessary.

Planning Phase

Planning begins with the selection of the memory compensation tools. As described in Chapter 2, a system is selected based on the capabilities of the client and a determination of what information needs to be tracked. During the selection of a memory compensation system, the long-term goals of the client, such as returning to work, are considered. However, during the planning phase of the implementation cycle, short-term goals that will allow the client to reach those long-term goals are defined. If achievable short-term goals are not defined, the foundation necessary to reach the larger goals is missing. It is not enough to just recommend memory compensation tools to the client and expect him or her to use them effectively. Many cycles of short-term goals that increase in complexity must be completed en route to reaching the long-term goals.

Establishing Short-Term Goals

The success of the treatment will depend heavily on good communication among the therapist, client, and support network. Input from all three are required to establish the treatment goals. It is usually easy for all involved parties to reach agreement concerning the long-term goals, such as returning to work. However, the path necessary to reach these goals is not usually obvious to everyone. Sometimes starting with small goals is frustrating to the client and support network. For instance, a family might be reluctant for the client to work only on properly taking medication when many other tasks (e.g., feeding a pet, paying bills, preparing meals) also need to be accomplished. Such frustration can be minimized with good communication. If the therapist is able to educate the client and support network about the treatment plan, in particular that small goals will lead to larger goals, then the groundwork for success is laid. If family members are able to see the value of starting with a limited but achievable goal, they are likely to provide the encouragement and support necessary for the treatment to progress.

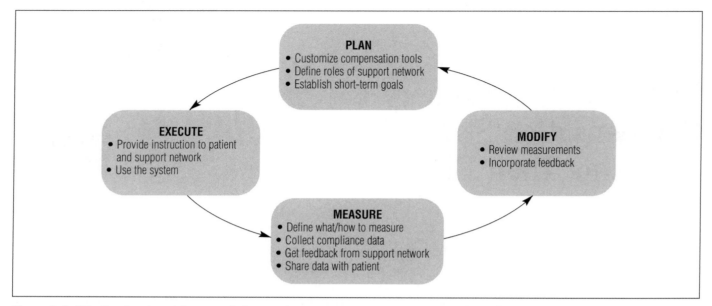

Figure 3.1. Effective treatment is an evolutionary process that requires repeated cycles of learning.

Because each client's situation is unique, there is no predefined list of short-term goals that are appropriate for all clients. Nevertheless, the basic idea that the early goals develop behaviors that enable reaching subsequent goals always applies. Some short-term goals to consider for each client are described below:

• *Having the tools available at all times.* Obviously if the needed memory compensation tools are not with the client, they're not being used. For example, if the therapist is working on a client's ability to use a checklist and he or she does not have it available when he or she needs it, then it will not be of benefit. From the start some clients have no problem keeping their memory compensation tools available, whereas others require extensive cuing from the therapist and support network.

• *Entering information immediately.* Most people who use personal organizers, forms, and checklists are able to wait for a convenient time to record information. For example, they may wait until the end of a conversation to write down the actions discussed. This is effective because they can rely on their memory. Most clients with memory impairment do not have that luxury. If they wait, they will likely forget to record many important things. For this reason they must develop the habit of entering information immediately upon receiving it. Most clients need substantial assistance in developing this habit.

• *Referring to the system frequently throughout the day.* Writing a note in a personal organizer is of no value if the organizer is never referenced. Many factors influence how frequently an organizer must be checked for it to be effective. Clients with extensive memory problems may need to reference their organizer hourly to record and retrieve information. Other clients may reference their organizer only three or four times a day. The frequency of use depends on the degree of the client's memory impairment and the responsibilities and actions that they are trying to accomplish.

• *Learning where to enter and retrieve information.* Without good organization, the chosen system will be ineffective. If, for instance, a client accidentally records an upcoming appointment in the daily pages of the organizer on the day that he or she arranges the appointment instead of the day that the appointment will take place, he or she will likely miss that appointment. Therefore, learning where to enter information and where to look to retrieve it later is necessary. A client may use many personalized items (e.g., checklists, maps, medical information) in his or her memory compensation system. Without a familiarity of where the information is stored, the client will be unable to retrieve it when needed.

• *Placing a check mark after completed tasks.* This is important because many clients with memory impairment are unable to remember completing tasks. The use of check marks, in both personal organizers and in checklists, gives the client a record of what he or she has completed if there is any question. It is important that the check marks be made immediately after the task is completed, and not before. It is very important to avoid instances in which a client places a check next to an item that he or she plans to complete very soon (e.g., taking medication). The client may become distracted, forget whether the task was completed, and then never complete the task because it has already been checked off.

• *Recording activities each hour.* Clients with severe memory impairment are often unable to recall what they have been doing from hour to hour. If they make a brief entry in their organizer describing their activities each hour, they will create a record that can give them a sense of continuity and accomplishment from day to day. Doing so also develops the necessary habit of consulting, retrieving, and recording information frequently throughout the day. In my experience, use of a watch with an hourly chime is always required to meet this goal.

• *Learning to write notes to self.* This means writing concise notes that contain sufficient detail to avoid confusion. If a client uses abbreviations, unfamiliar terms, or illegible writing that he or she has difficulty deciphering, the note will be useless. If the client records a name and phone number but forgets to include the purpose of the call, he or she may later remember to make the call but will not know why he or she is calling. Most clients need substantial assistance learning to write concise, meaningful notes.

Beginning with simple goals such as these provides a basis for achieving larger goals. Determination of short-term goals to use with each client should be a group effort guided by the therapist. All parties—client, therapist, and support network—should at least agree on the goal selection because they will all have to work together to ensure that the goals are reached.

Defining Roles of the Support Network

The role of the therapist is well defined: to guide the entire memory compensation training process. The role of the client also is clear. The client must be willing to participate in the treatment plan to the best of his or her ability. The members of the support network, however, often do not realize that they also play a vital role. They are essential in providing cues, modeling behaviors, providing feedback to the client when the therapist is not present, and reporting their observations to the therapist.

Whether the client is still in the hospital, at home, or trying to start back to work or school, the role played by the support network is essentially the same. It includes understanding the goals, being willing to provide cues and feedback to the client, and having an overall interest in seeing the client improve. Most of all, members of the support network must be aware that their

assistance is required. Good communication between the therapist and other care providers is necessary to develop this awareness.

The therapist should follow a few basic steps to clearly define the role of the support network in the client's treatment.

• *Identify the people that frequently interact with the client.* These people are usually family members, other medical staff, the client's supervisor and co-workers, and teachers if the client is in school. Identifying these individuals often requires visits to the client's home, school, or workplace.

• *Define expectations.* Unless the members of the support network clearly understand what is expected of them, the progress of the treatment will be delayed. Expectations that are directly linked to the goals of the treatment must be communicated. If the short-term goal is for the client to keep the personal organizer with him or her at all times, then family members or other medical staff must be willing to cue the client throughout the day. If they see that the client is leaving the room without his or her organizer, they need to know that it is their responsibility to remind the client to take the organizer along.

• *Get a commitment.* Once the expectations are outlined, a firm commitment from the members of the support network is vital. This commitment means more than just good intentions. Often family members or co-workers underestimate the amount of time and effort they are being asked to devote to the client's treatment. For instance, a family member may readily agree to always remind the client to carry his or her notebook. However, once the family member recognizes the tremendous vigilance required to constantly remind the client, he or she may become overwhelmed and lose sight of the therapy goals.

Situations like this occur often. The therapist not only must recognize such problems but also be willing to step in and work with the family member to remind him or her of the importance of his or her role in the client's treatment. Of course, the therapist needs to approach the family member with empathy. It is important for the therapist to let the family member know that the therapist understands the situation. It may seem hopeless and overwhelming to the family member at the time, but the therapist can remind him or her of the long-term goals. Once the client gets through the initial stages of treatment, the long-term goals will become clear and attainable, and it will get easier to see real, meaningful progress. The therapist needs, in a sense, to take on the role of a coach in getting everyone on the support team working together toward the common goal of a successful treatment outcome for the client.

As the treatment progresses, the roles of the members of the support network will change. Frequent interaction between the therapist and support network helps identify any changes and ensuing problems before the long-term goals of the client are jeopardized.

Customizing the Memory Compensation Tools

Once the short-term goals have been defined, a compensatory system that will facilitate meeting the goals must be organized:

• *Purchase the tools.* The previous chapter gives guidelines for selection of an appropriate system (see Figure 2.6). It is always helpful for the therapist to provide examples, such as copies of recommended personal organizer pages, to the client before the client purchases a system. It is sometimes even necessary to accompany the client to make the actual purchase. This ensures that the proper type of notebook or personal organizer, pillbox, watch, and so forth is obtained in a timely manner. I have learned this the hard way. More than once I have gotten off to a slow start with a client solely because it took several therapy sessions just to get the right tools in his or her hands.

• *Remove unneeded sections from the organizer.* Commercially available personal organizers usually include many sections (e.g., travel expenses, project tracking) that will never be used by the client with memory impairment. These sections should be removed from the organizer before beginning treatment because leaving them in may confuse the client.

• *Set up organizer sections that will be used.* Even though the initial focus of the treatment may not involve all sections of a personal organizer (or notebook) that will eventually be used, the therapist should set up all sections that the client can be expected to use eventually. For instance, the initial treatment emphasis may be only on the daily pages, but including other sections such as to-do lists, medical information, and a journal section will allow the client to become familiar with those sections early, before they are a focus of treatment. The details of setting up forms, procedures, and other personalized sections are discussed as follows in the execution phase.

Execution Phase

Once the proper memory compensation tools are selected, then the hard work of teaching the client and his or her support network how to use them begins. I call this the execution phase because at this point a plan is in

place—it just needs to be followed. That sounds simple enough, but the execution phase is always where the majority of everyone's (e.g., the client's, therapist's, support network's) time and effort are spent.

A former client of mine, whose case is detailed in Example D of Chapter 4, provides a good illustration of the importance of the execution phase. I started working with her approximately 1 year after she had stopped treatment with a different therapist following multiple brain surgeries for an aneurysm and a tumor. It was clear that she had been a very organized person before these surgeries. However, after the surgeries she had difficulty following through with even the most basic home management tasks (e.g., shopping, meal planning and preparation, bill paying). During a therapy session conducted in her home, I noticed an empty file box in her home office. When I asked her about it, she told me a story about how she came to purchase the file box. While working with her previous therapist, she expressed her frustration about not being able to keep her home bills organized. The therapist told her to get a file box, which was a good idea. The client took the file box to the next therapy session and asked what to do with it. She was told something like, "Just file your bills in there to keep them organized." That was it. One year later, the file box sat empty.

Although use of the memory compensation tools described in this manual seems like an easy thing for those of us without memory problems, it is often a different situation for people with memory impairment. It is easy to expect that a client will know what to do if you tell him or her to keep track of his or her appointments using a calendar. However, actually getting the client to do it properly is often a challenge.

In the sections that follow I provide guidelines for working with clients with memory impairment on how to use the memory compensation tools selected for them during the planning phase. Therapists approach memory compensation training from many angles. Some therapists may simply provide written instructions and expect the client to follow them. Others may provide no specific instructions and expect the client to learn through trial and error. I do not recommend either of these approaches. It is essential that the therapist take a more active role in the training. The approach that I find most effective is known as "errorless learning."

Using the Errorless-Learning Technique

Clients with memory impairment usually make very slow progress if they are allowed to make mistakes during the learning process. Depending on the severity of their memory problem, they may be unable to remember making a particular mistake. If given the opportunity, the client will continually repeat that same mistake. This leads to a situation in which the client encodes an incorrect procedure and actually learns to perform the given task incorrectly. In such cases it can be very difficult to then teach him or her the correct way to complete the task.

I have learned through experience that the most effective teaching approach with clients with memory impairment is to present instructions in a manner that makes it likely that they will perform the procedure correctly. This means providing step-by-step, detailed instructions that cannot be misinterpreted. This is a core aspect of the errorless-learning approach discussed in the "Introduction." Defining such instructions is a labor-intensive process that requires much interaction among the client, therapist, and support network.

A good example of the application of errorless learning involves the development and use of a checklist. The therapist first needs to learn in detail all of the steps necessary for the client to complete the activity. Next the therapist creates an initial checklist and works through it with the client. Revisions are made so that no steps are missed and each item is interpreted correctly. When complete, the checklist should provide an errorless procedure for the client to follow. If the client consistently uses the checklist when completing the activity, he or she will eventually encode the correct approach. In some cases he or she may progress to the point at which he or she no longer needs to use the checklist.

The errorless-learning approach can be applied to other areas besides checklists. Errorless learning is often helpful when teaching a client to correlate a watch chime with referencing a personal organizer. If all members of the support network ensure that the client immediately refers to the organizer when the watch chimes, then even a client with severe amnesia will eventually learn to do so consistently. During the learning stages of this behavior, it is very important that someone always be with the client to cue and physically assist with the procedure, maybe by actually opening the organizer to the proper page. As the client becomes more independent and less assistance is required, it is still necessary to monitor the client's compliance with the procedure and be ready to provide assistance if a mistake is about to be made.

As the therapist gains experience working on the implementation of memory compensation techniques, he or she will begin to anticipate areas in which individual clients are likely to have difficulty. By applying an errorless-learning approach to these areas, the therapist will enhance the client's ability to efficiently learn to compensate for his or her memory impairment.

Using a Wristwatch With Hourly Chime and Alarm

For any memory compensation tool to be effective, it must be referred to frequently. Many clients, especially those with moderate to severe memory impairment, are unable to keep track of time and often will forget to use their tools when needed. Clearly, a pillbox will not be effective if the client only happens upon it by chance. For such clients, a wristwatch with an alarm can provide an essential cue to take their medication at the prescribed time. Even clients with mild memory impairment may benefit from use of a watch with an hourly chime and alarm. The chime alerts them that it is the top of the hour, and the alarm can be set to alert them of approaching appointments.

Selecting a Suitable Watch. A brief visit to the watch counter of any department store will prove that many watches on the market include hourly chimes and alarms. They vary greatly in price and have a wide range of features, but not all of them are well suited for use by clients with memory impairment. It is usually best for the therapist to assist the family and client in the purchase of the watch. When selecting a watch, the following things should be considered:

- *Ease of use.* Many clients are attracted to wristwatches that have many features. Digital watches with calculators, altimeters, and so forth are common. Each additional feature not only increases the price of the watch, it also makes the watch more complicated to use. I suggest that watches with only basic features, including the time, day and date, hourly chime, alarm, and stopwatch, be used with most clients.

- *Loud chime with double beep.* For the watch to be effective, the client must be able to hear the sound of the chime even in a noisy, distracting environment. The tone and volume of watch chimes vary considerably and are neither specific nor standardized by the manufacturer. It is therefore usually necessary to compare several different models at the store. It is strongly recommended that the chime consist of a double beep.

A small percentage of my clients are unable to hear even the loudest watch chimes. This could be because of hearing problems or because they work in a particularly noisy environment. In those cases I have recommended watches with a vibration feature in addition to the audible alarm. Most department stores do not carry vibration watches, but they can be ordered through companies that specialize in equipment for people with hearing impairments.

• *Simultaneous time and date display.* Many digital watches have separate displays for the day and date, requiring the wearer to press a button to view one or the other. Because most clients with memory impairment will frequently need to check both date and time together, watches with a simultaneous display of date, day of the week, and time of day are recommended.

• *Symbols for alarm and chime.* Most digital watches have an alarm symbol that is visible in the normal time mode, but many do not have a similar symbol for the chime. It is important that the client, therapist, or member of the support network be able to confirm with a quick look at the watch that the chime is properly set to sound each hour.

Setting Instructions for Watch Use. Most clients cannot learn to use the needed features of a watch without assistance. The manufacturer's operation instructions included with watches are usually written in a manner that is confusing to clients with memory impairment. The recommended approach is for the therapist to provide simplified instructions tailored for client use. Step-by-step instructions for the functions frequently used by the client, such as setting the watch to chime

each hour and setting and turning off the alarm, should be given.

An example of watch instructions that I supply to my clients with memory impairment is given in Figure 3.2. It is important that the instructions be concise and easy to follow so that the client is not likely to make mistakes when using the watch.

Of course, it is not enough to provide the instructions and expect the client to follow them without problems. I often spend the majority of one or two therapy sessions teaching the client to properly use the watch. Once in a while I have a client who is very familiar with using a digital watch and needs very little instruction. However, most of the time it is necessary to repeat the procedure of setting and re-setting the alarm many times (as many as 10–20 times) during those initial sessions. I will ask the client to set the watch alarm to sound in 5 minutes. I closely monitor him or her while he or she follows the instructions to set the alarm and intervene if he or she is about to make a mistake. Once the alarm is set, we will work on something else until it sounds. Then we follow the procedure to turn off the alarm and then reset the alarm to sound again in 5 minutes.

Thus, in accordance with the errorless-learning technique, I supply the client with detailed, step-by-step

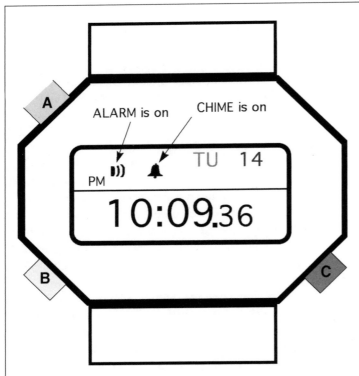

FUNCTIONS
CHIME—goes off on the hour
ALARM—goes off for the time that it is set

CHIME INSTRUCTIONS ("chime" should always be on)
1. Press button **B** until the letters "AL" are displayed.
2. Press button **C** to rotate through "alarm" and "chime" symbols, until only the "chime" symbol is showing.
3. Press button **B** *once* to return to normal time mode.
4. The chime is now set.

ALARM INSTRUCTIONS
1. Press button **B** until the letters "AL" are displayed.
2. Press button **A** to begin alarm setting procedure (hour should be flashing).
3. Press button **C** to advance hours. The letters PM will appear in the upper-left-hand corner if the alarm is to be set for a PM time.
4. Press button **A** to start next number flashing. Use button **C** to advance numbers.
5. Press button **A** once the alarm time is set.
6. Press button **B** to return to normal display. The alarm is now set and armed. The "alarm" ■)) symbol should be showing.

TO TURN OFF THE ALARM
1. Press button **B** until the letters "AL" are displayed.
2. Press button **C** to rotate through "alarm" and "chime" symbols, until only the "chime" symbol is showing.
3. Press button **B** *once* to return to normal time mode.
4. The alarm is now turned off and the hourly chime is left on.

Figure 3.2. Watch instructions.

instructions, I guide the client through the instructions to ensure that they are followed correctly, and I anticipate and prevent the client from making mistakes. Most clients need to use the instructions for only a short time before becoming independent with the watch alarm procedures.

Learning to Use a Personal Organizer

Nearly every client whom I see eventually uses some type of a personal organizer. As discussed in Chapter 2, personal organizers range in complexity from a simple binder or notebook to complex daily planners. Some suggested techniques to begin use of the personal organizer elements are outlined in the sections that follow. Approaches for working with a variety of clients who have a wide range of needs and capabilities are discussed. It is up to the therapist to choose from the following methods those that most appropriately address the client's unique situation.

Keeping the Organizer in Possession at All Times. It seems obvious, but the first and most important step in using a personal organizer is making sure that the organizer is always available to the client. Some clients automatically keep their organizer with them at all times. For various reasons, other clients have difficulty with this. Clients with severe memory problems may forget that they even have an organizer, let alone where they last left it. Some strategies that are useful in ensuring that the organizer is available at all times are described below:

• *Train the support network.* All members of the support network must be trained to cue the client to keep the organizer in his or her possession. This means that the members of the support network must be observant and diligent in reminding the client.

• *Identify a prominent place for keeping the organizer.* Many clients are disorganized and do not have a consistent place where they keep their organizer. Identifying a place at home on the kitchen counter or dining table where the organizer is always kept is advised. The place should be highly visible so that the client will see it frequently throughout the day and notice it when leaving the house. There should be enough space to have the book open so that it can be used without moving it. Similar considerations should be given if the client will use the organizer at work or school.

• *Place notes or placards where they cannot be overlooked.* Notes placed on a door exiting the house or on the steering wheel of a car can be used to ensure that a client remembers the organizer. It is, of course, com-pletely useless to place such reminders in the organizer itself.

Consulting the Organizer Regularly. Ensuring that the client has the organizer in his or her possession does not automatically mean that it will be of any use to the client. The next step is to teach the client to refer to it frequently. This step is almost automatic for people without memory impairment. I say "almost" because even those of us without memory impairment sometimes miss appointments despite having them correctly entered in our organizers. Such things can happen to any of us, but a client with memory impairment is particularly susceptible.

If I have an appointment on a Tuesday, I may check my organizer early Tuesday morning to confirm the time. Later in the day I may need to reconfirm the time if I have any doubts. I think this is the way that most of us use our organizers. However, a client with memory impairment may check the organizer early Tuesday morning and "discover" that he or she has an appointment that day at 3:30 p.m. If the next time the client looks at the organizer is 6:00 p.m., then he or she most likely will have missed the appointment. Situations such as this are common, and the most effective way to avoid them is to ensure that the client refers to the organizer frequently.

• *Consulting the organizer every hour.* Some clients need to check their organizer every hour. An example is a client with severe amnesia who cannot remember what he or she has done or needs to do from hour to hour. Another example is a client with only mild memory deficits but who has extensive responsibilities with many activities to track each day. In either case, a watch with an hourly chime must be used to prompt the client to refer to the organizer. The objective is to teach the client to associate the sound of the chime with the act of referring to the organizer to enter and retrieve information. Clients with mild impairment typically do not require much training to learn this procedure.

On the other hand, months of intensive training may be required for clients with severe memory impairment. To ensure that the association is made, members of the support network must be assigned the role of immediately cuing the client to refer to the book each hour when the chime sounds. To be effective, the cue must be provided in a manner that does not allow the client to become confused about the association between the chime and organizer. For example, when the chime sounds, asking the client what he or she should do is likely to cause him or her to guess and give incorrect answers. The concept of referring to the book at the sound of the chime will be lost. A better approach is to immediately tell the client what to do and to help him or her do it so that he or she will not have the opportunity to make a mistake.

This is another example of the errorless-learning technique. The person providing the cues must anticipate that the chime will sound so that the cue can be given quickly. The person also must make sure that the organizer is within easy reach.

• *Consulting the organizer at predefined times.* For clients with mild impairment who need to refer to the organizer only three or four times each day, it is usually best to establish a routine of consulting the organizer at fixed times associated with other routine activities such as meals. By consulting the organizer early in the day (e.g., at breakfast), a reminder of that day's events is given. Consultation late in the day (e.g., at bedtime) allows the client to prepare for the next day's activities.

• *Consulting the organizer at variable times.* Because many activities do not occur on the hour or at other predefined times throughout the day, it is often necessary to use a watch with an alarm that can be easily set for any time as a reminder to consult the organizer. An important consideration is that the alarm must sometimes be set early to allow travel time to an appointment or event. Such considerations are not always obvious to clients with memory impairment.

Using the Daily Pages

The daily pages are one of the most frequently used sections of a personal organizer. Most people use the daily pages for planning upcoming events. However, clients with severe impairment also may use them to keep a record of their activities throughout each day.

Entering Information

• *Where to enter information.* The entries in the daily pages must be made in a consistent, organized manner. It is impossible to describe all of the effective ways in which data can be recorded. However, in all cases it is important that entries are placed near the corresponding time that the action will occur.

Sometimes clients, especially those with severe memory impairment, need help finding the correct page to make an entry. Most personal organization systems come with a page marker that is a useful guide to rapidly accessing the correct page. Although most clients are able to quickly understand the purpose of the page marker, teaching the client to properly use it is sometimes necessary. The client must develop the habit of moving the marker ahead at a consistent time each day, either at the end of the day or first thing in the morning.

He or she also must learn to verify, by checking a calendar or watch with the date, that he or she has moved the marker to the proper day. If the organizer being used does not include a page marker, then a substitute, such as a paper clip attached to the top of the page, should be used. It is sometimes necessary, especially early in treatment, to provide cues for the client to use the page marker. Finding the location on the page that corresponds to the correct time of day may require an additional cue.

It seems obvious that a reminder for an action to be completed at 9:00 a.m. should be placed on the page at the 9:00 a.m. time slot, but many clients have difficulty with this. They may enter information without regard to the time or day that the action should occur. An example is a client who on Wednesday arranges for a Friday appointment but enters the appointment information on Wednesday's page. The best method of working with clients on this issue is to repeatedly demonstrate the correct method of entering information and to provide many opportunities for the client to practice. The therapist will be able to assist the client when entries are made during therapy sessions. However, the therapist also must train the members of the support network because most entries will probably need to be made outside therapy sessions, when they are the only ones available to provide assistance.

• *When to enter information.* Information must be entered as soon as it is received. Because clients with memory impairment are easily distracted, any delay can cause them to completely forget to make the entry. Again, the most effective method of teaching the client is to provide many opportunities to practice both during and outside therapy sessions. Members of the support network must be taught to cue the client to make the entry promptly. For example, a work supervisor who informs the client of a meeting also should ensure that the client enters this information in the organizer and provide a cue if needed.

• *Writing legible, concise notes.* The daily pages in most organizers have only limited space to write notes. Thus, the entries must be short and clearly written to be effective. Because of cognitive, language, and physical impairments, clients often have difficulty writing short, meaningful, and legible notes.

Providing concrete examples for the client is the most practical method of developing this skill. In initial treatment sessions I may dictate to the client appropriate notes for various situations. Most notes must include a place and topic and need to be entered in the appropriate time slot. For instance, if the client has an upcoming appointment at 2:30 p.m. on Thursday for math tutoring, I would instruct him or her to enter the note "Meet Kent for math tutoring in library" in the 2:30 p.m. time slot on Thursday's page. If any vital information is not recorded, the note will be of little use. If, for instance, the topic "math tutoring" is left out of the note, the client may forget to bring his or her math book to the meeting.

Some clients have difficulty reading their own writing. In many cases, this is because the client is trying to write too quickly, and making a suggestion to slow down is enough to resolve this. Sometimes the client must be encouraged to print as a means of slowing down. Through the use of customized rubber stamps, clients who cannot write legibly can achieve limited use of the daily pages. Rubber stamps with preprinted notes for routine tasks, such as taking medication, will allow the client to make legible entries for those tasks.

Clients may have difficulty summarizing complex information into a concise entry. This is especially true if the client has language difficulties or a decreased speed of information processing. The therapist must make members of the support network aware of such problems and instruct them on effective approaches. The information given must be specific and concise. The client must understand the information and what actions he or she is expected to take. Clients who do not understand the information must feel comfortable asking for clarification. It often is best to have the client repeat the information back to the person giving it to confirm that it was correctly understood. It also is useful to have the person giving the information review the entry made by the client in the organizer.

In my caseload nearly all of the clients are at a level in which they are able to learn to write clear notes in their daily pages. However, there are cases in which the client's cognitive, language, and physical deficits render him or her completely unable to use the daily pages. In such situations, it may be necessary for the client to rely entirely on checklists and customized forms to achieve any degree of functional independence.

Retrieving Information

• *Scanning for information.* Many clients are impulsive and do not take the time to completely read the notes that they have made. They also may look at the wrong time of day or reference the wrong page of the organizer.

Many opportunities for practice are usually required before an impulsive client learns to thoroughly read the notes in the organizer. The first step is to ensure that the client refers to the correct time and date

on the daily pages. The page marker described earlier helps with this, but the client also must learn to verify the correct time slot. This means that the client must correlate the time of day with the entries made in the organizer.

The next step is to ensure that the client completely reads the entries on the daily pages so that actions that must be completed are not overlooked. The best way to work on this is to thoroughly review the daily pages during therapy sessions. The therapist might ask the client what tasks need to be completed at a specific time. The client should read back the entire entry to the therapist. Often the entry at a specific time will have multiple steps. A common mistake is for the client to read only the first part of the entry. Repeated practice, often facilitated through assignments given by the therapist, is usually needed to teach the client to accurately read the entries. As with other procedures it is important for the client to also practice this skill outside the therapy sessions. And, as usual, the assistance of the members of the support network is essential.

• *Marking completed tasks.* Clients must learn to mark completed tasks immediately after completion and not before. Many clients will learn this with little instruction, but some will always make mistakes unless it is a primary focus early in the treatment. Some clients will correctly read an entry and then mark it as completed because they intend to perform the task soon. If distracted, they may forget to complete the task. When they refer back to their organizer they see the check mark and assume the task has been completed. This can be a particularly serious problem if they are relying on their organizer as a cue to take their medication or perform child care.

The only way to tell for sure if the client has this problem is to observe him or her completing tasks entered in the organizer. The therapist or a member of the support network must be present to provide instruction when the client is learning to properly mark completed tasks. If they are not allowed to make mistakes, most clients will quickly learn to properly mark their completed tasks.

At every therapy session I review the client's daily pages with him or her in detail. I go through all entries not only on the present page but also back to the last therapy session and forward a couple of weeks. I check that clear and concise notes are entered in the correct locations and that the completed tasks have a check mark next to them. This review gives me an indication of problem areas that should be the focus of treatment. In cases in which past tasks have not been completed, the tasks are moved forward to a future page if appropriate.

Using the Month-in-a-View Planning Calendar

The month-in-a-view calendar is used to plan and track activities on a long-term scale. Information recorded in this section is often transferred to the daily pages if specific actions must be completed. Most clients have little difficulty understanding the purpose of these pages because many have used similar calendars before. The most common problem is that clients will not remember to consistently review this section.

Determining What Information Belongs. In general, information regarding infrequent or nonroutine events is recorded in the month-in-a-view calendar. Special occasions such as birthdays, anniversaries, vacations, and family gatherings are usually first recorded in this section and later transferred to the daily pages. Many clients also record significant financial information such as paydays or dates when bills are due. Nonroutine home management chores such as changing the oil in a car or fertilizing plants also may be listed.

Another reason that the month-in-a-view calendar is important is that an entire year, or even 2 years, of monthly calendar pages can easily be included in the organizer, whereas it is usually impractical to include more than about 6 months of daily pages. If an entry regarding a task that will occur many months in the future must be made, the calendar pages provide a location. Later, once the required daily pages are loaded into the organizer, such an entry must be transferred to the correct daily page.

Entering Information. As with all sections of the organizer, the information entered in the monthly calendar must be organized and concise to be useful. Because the space for entries on these pages is very limited, the entries made will not contain as much detail as those in the daily pages. Early in the treatment, the therapist may ask the client to bring to therapy a list of pertinent dates (e.g., birthdays) that the client needs to remember and then assist the client with properly entering that information in the monthly pages. Once that initial information is entered, it provides a foundation that the client can build on as needed.

It also is important that members of the support network be aware of this section so that they will provide cues to the client to make entries when appropriate. In addition, some clients will have difficulty writing clearly in the limited space provided, and members of the support network may need to enter the information for them.

Remembering to Review the Calendar. Because this section is not referenced as often as the daily pages, some clients may neglect to reference it at all. To avoid this problem it is important that the monthly calendar, and all other sections of the organizer, be reviewed during each therapy session. Another approach is to include reminder notes in the daily pages. Such notes may be placed at the beginning or end of each week or month. This helps the client develop the habit of reviewing these pages on a regular basis.

Transferring Information to the Daily Pages. If an item entered in the month-in-a-view calendar requires an action by the client on a specific day, then the information must be transferred to the appropriate day in the daily pages. If, for example, an appointment is made 6 months in advance and the daily pages for the date of the appointment are not in the organizer, that appointment will be recorded on the monthly calendar. Once the daily page corresponding to the appointment date is available, the information must be transferred. Each time new daily pages are added to the organizer, the monthly calendar pages should be thoroughly reviewed to ensure that all necessary information is transferred.

The transfer of information to the daily pages is slightly more complicated when the client must perform activities before the event listed in the monthly calendar. An example is a student who records in his monthly calendar that a term paper is due on a certain date. Because term papers are rarely completed in one day, the student must not only transfer the due date to the daily pages, but also make an entry on the date he or she will begin working on the paper. Similar considerations must be made for occasions such as birthdays and anniversaries when a card or gift must be purchased in advance.

Using To-Do Lists

To-do lists provide a medium- to long-range planning tool for activities that do not have to be completed on a particular day or at a specific hour. As with the month-in-a-view calendar, most clients have little difficulty understanding the purpose of to-do lists but may forget to refer to them regularly. Activities such as cleaning out a closet that need to be completed but do not have a specific deadline should be included on to-do lists.

The process used for entering information on a to-do list is similar to that used for the month-in-a-view calendar. Because most clients have used such lists in the past, they usually are able to make entries after only minimal instruction. Again, it is important that the members of the support network are aware of this section and cue the client to include items on the to-do list when appropriate. As with the monthly calendar pages, the to-do list is not referenced as often as the daily pages, and some clients forget to reference it at all. Reminder notes in the daily pages are an effective method of teaching the client to review the to-do list consistently.

All to-do lists should include a means of indicating when a task has been completed or transferred to the daily pages. Once a particular date or time is chosen for completing an item on the to-do list, that information must be transferred to the appropriate daily page. Of course, if the task is completed immediately there is no need to transfer it to the daily pages. If for some reason the task is not completed as planned in the daily pages, it will either need to be reentered on the to-do list or moved forward in the daily pages.

I believe that the to-do list format should be as simple as possible. I recommend having only three columns: one for the date the entry is made, one describing the task, and one for the date of completion or transfer to the daily pages. Figure 2.3 shows an example of a typical to-do list format I use with my clients.

Using Forms, Checklists, and Procedures

Forms, checklists, and procedures are custom pages designed to assist the client with performing, recording, and tracking activities. Forms provide a practical means for clients to accumulate and summarize information on a particular topic. They are used when the details of the activity are not yet fully defined. For example, a client taking classes may use a form to keep track of homework assignments given during the semester. At the beginning of the semester, the student does not know what assignments will be given, only that there will be assignments. The form could provide a template for recording the details of each assignment and its due date.

Checklists, procedures, and procedural checklists, on the other hand, are used when the details of the activity are fully defined. Checklists provide a structured outline for repeated activities and help ensure that the activities are completed correctly each time. A pilot's preflight checklist, as mentioned earlier, is a good example of a procedural checklist.

A standard checklist is simply a list of tasks that need to be completed on a repeating basis. For example a client might have a basic checklist that he or she uses each day, including items such as "take medication,"

"make bed," "wash dishes," "feed the cat." The order that the items are listed does not really matter.

If, however, the client needs more direction to complete an item, he or she also may need a procedural checklist. For example, if the client is having difficulty sequencing the steps involved in taking his or her medication, the procedural checklist might include the following:

• Get glass of water.
• Open pillbox to correct day (verify with calendar).
• Take pills.
• Close pillbox.

Of course, in a procedural checklist the order is very important. If the steps are not done in sequence, then there will be problems.

Despite their differences, the process for developing forms, checklists, and procedures is very similar.

Developing Customized Forms. Forms are most useful when the client needs to frequently refer to the information being tracked and has difficulty using the daily pages for this purpose. An example is a client who has several projects at work. Keeping track of all of them on the daily pages may be too confusing. Such a client might benefit from a separate form to track the details of each project.

The first thing I do when developing a customized form with a client is to meet with the client to learn what he or she needs to accomplish with the form. Once the needs of the client are determined, it is then my job to define an initial form that will facilitate meeting those needs. I cannot recall a single case in which my initial form was perfect; there is always some amount of revision required. The single most important aspect of form creation is making revisions based on feedback from the client and support network. As the client begins to use the form, certain modifications that will make it more effective will become clear. The modifications may be as simple as increasing the size of the area for writing notes or making entries. In other cases, the therapist may determine that additional items need to be included on the form.

Developing Checklists and Procedures. Because the purpose of a checklist is to ensure consistency in the completion of an activity, it is necessary for the therapist to learn the minute details of the activity to create a useful checklist. Development of detailed checklists is a time-consuming process; therefore, only activities that the client expects to repeat often are good candidates for checklists. It is important to get input and agreement from both the client and members of the support network when determining what activities to target.

When developing a procedural checklist, the details of the task, such as which file cabinet contains the needed folders, can be learned only if the therapist observes the client attempting to complete the task. This means that the therapist must leave the clinic and work with the client in the environment in which the task will be completed. Interaction with the support network also is necessary to ensure that no steps are overlooked. If the client knew all of the details to include, he or she most likely would not need the procedural checklist in the first place.

The most effective means of developing a checklist is by trial and error. Even experienced therapists who have carefully observed the client's activities and have a clear understanding of the steps involved in the tasks will not make a perfect checklist on the first try. It is best to quickly generate the first draft of the checklist and observe the client using it. Through observation the needed revisions to the checklist will be apparent. Some items on the checklist may need rewording so that the client can understand them. Steps may have been left off or described with insufficient detail. Some steps may be too long and need to be divided into multiple substeps. This trial-and-error process may include multiple iterations over several days or weeks before a checklist that allows the client to independently complete the activity is defined.

Including Forms, Checklists, and Procedures in the Organizer. Because the client must be able to quickly locate needed forms and checklists, it is usually best to provide a separate section in the organizer for them. It also is helpful to use tabs or color coding to highlight particular forms and checklists or to group them by category. If the same checklist is used repeatedly, it is either necessary for the client to have multiple copies available or to place the checklist in a plastic sleeve and use an erasable marker. In some cases, clients who use many forms and checklists may require a separate book for them.

Cross-Referencing to Other Organizer Sections. Many times items included in forms and checklists require action on a specific date. For example, a student using a form to track homework assignments may need to reference that form in the daily pages of his or her organizer to ensure that the assignment is not forgotten. Other items might be cross-referenced to different forms or to-do lists.

To effectively use forms and checklists, the client must learn to frequently review them and transfer the necessary information to other sections of the organizer. Teaching the client to do this usually requires exten-

sive training. It is recommended that the therapist review all sections of the personal organizer with the client regularly to promote cross-referencing. In this way, the process for using a form or checklist is similar to that for a monthly calendar or to-do list. The goal is for the client to develop the habit of regularly reviewing the forms and checklists in the organizer and transferring pertinent information to other sections.

Interacting With the Support Network. It is important to ensure that the client's support network is aware of and understands the purpose of the forms and checklists that the client has available. This is best accomplished through frequent therapist interaction with the client's support network. It also is vital that the members of the support network fully understand their role in helping the client use forms and checklists. Many times the support network not only suggests topics for forms and checklists but also helps define the details included and cues the client about their use.

Many clients who have experienced brain injury will never be fully independent. The degree to which they achieve independence often depends heavily on the abilities of their support network. For this reason it is important to teach the support network the process of developing forms and checklists. If, for example, a client moves to a new house, the details in a procedural checklist related to housecleaning will certainly change. If the support network is able to create a new checklist applicable to the new environment, a certain degree of independence is maintained. In such a case, the client is able to adapt to a new situation without a therapist's intervention.

Using All Parts of the System Together

Daily pages, month-in-a-view calendars, to-do lists, and customized forms and checklists are all items that can be included in a personal organizer. Other memory compensation tools such as those described in Chapter 2 (e.g., wristwatch, pillbox, timer, dry-erase board) clearly do not fit in an organizer but are frequently used in conjunction with one. The following example illustrates how these tools can work together:

> A client's **wristwatch chime** is set to sound on the hour, cuing him to reference his **organizer**. In the **daily pages** for that hour he finds a note indicating that it is time to take his medication. He then goes to his **pillbox** (which is always in a **designated place**) and takes the correct pills. Only after the pills are taken does he place a **checkmark in the daily page** entry to mark the task as completed.

There are, of course, thousands of ways that these tools can work together to complete the different tasks that each client must perform. It is a therapist's job to determine what problems the client is encountering as he or she attempts to complete a task. Thus, the therapist must develop a thorough understanding of not only the client's deficits but also the details of the task. Direct observation is almost always the most efficient way to develop that understanding. Once the therapist has observed the client, then he or she will be able to select the memory compensation tools (and combinations thereof) that are likely to be of help.

Practicing Using Memory Compensation Tools

We've all heard the saying "practice makes perfect." We know from personal experience that when learning something new—for instance, a new language or sport—the initial instructions are not enough. To become fluent in a language or adept at a sport, practice is essential. This also is true for memory compensation training. Without ample opportunities to practice using memory compensation tools, the client will never become proficient with them.

Each client's unique situation determines the number of opportunities that he or she will have to use his or her memory compensation tools each day. A client who has returned to work and has many responsibilities may need to refer to his or her organizer every hour to schedule and attend meetings or follow up on assignments. Purely by the nature of his or her own situation, he or she will have many opportunities to use his or her compensation tools.

On the other hand, a client who has been recently discharged from in-patient rehabilitation is not likely to have many responsibilities or tasks to complete. One common situation is a client who needs to learn to use an organizer with daily pages but has only limited activities to track each day. If he or she opens the organizer, most of the pages will be blank. Such a client will benefit from additional assignments designed to provide opportunities for practice using his or her organizer. During therapy sessions I will assign simple, concrete tasks for this type of client to complete each day. For example, I may ask the client to call my voice mail at 10:00 a.m. and leave a message about the current weather. This gives the client the opportunity to enter a clear and concise note in the proper location on the daily page, refer to the note at a specific time, complete the task, and mark it as completed. I may assign three or four such tasks each day (including weekends). Depending on how successful the client is at completing these simple tasks, I will be able to tell what area to focus on in therapy.

The example just given focuses on using daily pages but can be generalized to using forms, checklists, a watch alarm, or any of the other memory compensation tools. The assignments need to be straightforward and measurable, as is discussed in the next section. Some practical examples of how I have worked with my clients to provide opportunities for them to practice using their memory compensation tools are given in Chapter 4.

Measurement Phase

Once goals have been set and execution of a treatment plan is under way, it is essential that a means of measuring progress be established. Most clients progress slowly, and without an objective measurement tool it is very difficult to quantify the level of their improvement. The data collected provides concrete information to the therapist, client, and support network that helps define where treatment efforts should be concentrated.

Starting With Short-Term Goals

It seems obvious that the items to be measured should support the goals of the treatment plan. I always recommend an approach that begins with small, short-term goals that establish a foundation for achieving the larger long-term goals of the treatment. For instance, reaching the long-term goal of independent organizer use might start with the short-term goal of having the organizer available at all times. Several other short-term goals related to independent personal organizer use were described in detail earlier in the section on the planning phase.

Once the therapist becomes familiar with the client's deficits, it is likely that many possible things to measure will become evident. However, if the measurement process is too complicated, it is likely that the therapist will not get the necessary participation of the client and support network. Therefore, it is recommended that only 1 or 2 items be measured at a time. Although the therapist should take the lead in defining them, there must be communication and participation among all parties concerning the objective of the measurements. By selecting items that are not too complicated and are achievable, the client will be able to observe his or her own progress. This creates an encouraging environment in which the client and support network are likely to see the value of the treatment and continue participation. The therapist must be careful to select items that are not too advanced for the client's abilities. If the client is unable to make progress on the measured items, he or she will become frustrated and may lose motivation to continue.

The bottom line is that the therapist should not overwhelm the client and support network with assignments to measure progress. If the client and support network feel that they are spending too much time measuring progress and not enough time actually using the memory compensation tools, they may begin to consider the entire process as more of a nuisance than a benefit.

Collecting Compliance Data

To objectively assess a client's progress toward established goals, a considerable amount of data collection is usually required. The therapist usually gathers some of the data during sessions with the client. However, because the client spends most of his or her time outside therapy sessions, the majority of the data will be gathered by members of the support network. It is not advised to ask the client to gather his or her own compliance data. For various reasons, data gathered by the client are usually not reliable.

Defining a Data Collection Procedure. After 1 or 2 items to measure have been identified, the next step is to set up a procedure for collecting the data. This usually begins with the creation of a customized tracking form that provides a template for data collection. For reasons described earlier, it is important that the tracking form and the entire data collection procedure be as simple as possible. Four basic categories that need to be included on all forms are described below:

1. *Date/Time.* To keep track of the client's progress, it is always necessary to record the date, and often the time, that the data were collected. This information is needed to examine trends in the client's performance over specific time intervals (e.g., weeks or months).

2. *Compliance.* The percentage of items that the client successfully completed is usually what is measured. The item should be in the form of a clear, specific "yes/no" question. For instance, if the goal is for the client to carry the organizer at all times, the question might be "Does Nancy have her organizer with her?" Avoid vague questions such as "Is Nancy using the organizer?"

3. *Comments.* In many instances a simple "yes" or "no" response may not be enough to fully describe the client's ability to successfully complete the task. A space to record observations often helps to more thoroughly describe the data being collected. For instance, if a client's ability to keep the organizer with him or her is being tracked on an hourly basis, and the client has left

the organizer at home, a series of "no" responses for the entire day will be indistinguishable from the series of "no" responses that would result from a case in which the client has repeatedly left the organizer behind throughout the day. A comment indicating that the client left the organizer at home will make the data more meaningful.

4. *Signature.* Many times questions arise concerning the compliance data that have been gathered. Often the therapist must contact the person who made an entry to gain a better understanding of the circumstances regarding the entry. For this reason it is important that each person recording data sign or initial his or her entries.

As mentioned earlier, most of the data are gathered outside therapy sessions. For this reason the therapist must rely on the support network for most of the data collection, and guidelines for the data collection process must be communicated. Common issues to discuss include the frequency of making entries in the tracking form, the interpretation of the yes/no question on the form, and the use of the comments category.

Frequency of data collection. The frequency of data collection depends on the item being measured and the individual situation of the client. Once an item to measure is selected, the therapist should be able to predict how often the client is likely to have the opportunity to perform the task. For example, if the item being measured is the client's compliance with referring to the organizer at the sound of the hourly chime, there should be more than 10 opportunities each day. Other items, such as independent use of the watch alarm (not hourly chime) for upcoming appointments might occur only a few times a week.

It also is necessary to consider when members of the support network are available to record the data. In the hourly chime example mentioned earlier, the client might be awake 16 hours each day but in the presence of the therapist or members of the support network only 12 of those hours, and maybe fewer on weekends. This means that 12 opportunities for data collection occur each weekday.

The task being measured should be defined such that at least 2 or 3 opportunities for measurement occur each day. This minimum ensures that there will be sufficient data collected to track progress on at least a weekly basis and also provides sufficient opportunities for most clients to develop a habit of successfully completing the task. In many instances, such as the watch alarm example above, the therapist must generate assignments to provide the client with the needed opportunities to perform the task.

Interpretation of the yes–no question. Clear guidelines for the response to the yes–no question must be communicated by the therapist to all members of the support network recording data. Even very simple yes–no questions often do not have "black-or-white" answers. Many times a significant gray area exists. The example question given earlier, "Does Nancy have her organizer with her?" seems clear and easy to answer. If, however, Nancy arrives at a therapy session without her organizer and soon remembers to go get it, how should the question be answered? In such situations it is recommended that a "no" response regarding compliance be recorded. The general rule is that if it's not 100% "yes," then it is "no." The client may argue that this is not fair, but it is the only way to obtain unequivocal data, and more importantly, to ensure that the client learns the proper behavior.

Use of comments. In the example just given, a "no" response and a brief comment indicating that the client immediately remembered to get the organizer would fully describe the situation. Members of the support network should be encouraged to write comments that explain their entries or describe what they have observed whenever they feel it is appropriate. Too many comments are better than not enough.

A sample tracking form that includes all of the categories discussed above, and a few others, is included in Figure 3.3. In this form, several examples are given of memory assignments provided by the therapist to give the client opportunities to practice using the organizer.

If the items being tracked relate to personal organizer use, it is usually easiest to keep the tracking form in the back of the client's organizer. Assuming that the organizer is with the client, this will make the form available to all members of the support network when they need to record data. It is not recommended to provide each member of the support network with a separate tracking form. If everyone uses the same form, all of the data will be sequentially ordered and accessible in one place.

Even though the tracking form should be kept in the organizer, it is not recommended that the client make entries to the form or refer to it to determine what activities need to be completed. The other sections of the organizer, usually the daily pages, should be used by the client for this purpose. The intent of the tracking form is to record how well the client is using the organizer, not to provide a substitute for using the other sections of the organizer.

The examples discussed earlier focused on a client learning to use a personal organizer. If the client is learning to use one of the other memory compensation tools (e.g., pillbox, dry-erase board, wristwatch), a similar measurement approach is recommended.

Summarizing and Sharing Data With Client and Support Network. Many therapists are not accustomed

Date Assigned	Assigned by	Task	Date Due	Accurate Y	Accurate N	Comments	Initials
10/3	D.C.	Tell Mom about soccer team party	10/4	–			J.a.
10/3	S.K.	Ask Maria where to get word search books	10/5		–	Note to self not clear	M.M.
10/4	S.K.	Call Sue at 9 a.m. Saturday	10/6		–	Not on time	S.K.
10/4	D.C.	Bring in reading homework	10/5	–			D.C.
10/4	S.K.	Ask Dennis if he likes Michael Jackson	10/5	–			D.C.
10/4	S.K.	Tell Sue answer to above at 10 a.m. Tuesday	10/9		–	Not on time	S.K.
10/4	L.M.	Ask Mom who will pick me up Friday	10/5	–			L.M.
10/4	L.M.	Write answer to above on Friday's page	10/5	–			L.M.
10/5	S.K.	At 11 a.m. Monday set watch alarm for 11:20 a.m.	10/8	–			M.M.
10/5	S.K.	At 11:20 a.m., ask Dennis where his next vacation will be	10/8	–			D.C.
10/5	S.K.	At 3 p.m. tell Sue answer to above question	10/8		–	Required cue to give information	S.K.

Figure 3.3. Tracking sheet for personal organizer assignments.

to sharing their notes with clients. The development and implementation of memory compensation training is a group effort that includes the therapist, the client, and the client's support network. Because the participation of all parties is vital to the success of the treatment, the data that is used to assess the client's progress should be shared regularly with all participants. Sharing concrete information about the client's progress helps all parties involved develop a realistic appraisal of the client's abilities and weaknesses. This encourages acceptance of therapy goals, fosters a team atmosphere, and promotes an environment of continued participation.

The compliance data should be summarized by the therapist before sharing it with the client and support network. Usually a percentage of compliance is calculated based on the data gathered. Depending on the frequency of data collection, as discussed earlier, the percentage of compliance should be calculated daily or weekly. Waiting until the end of the month is usually not effective in providing useful feedback. When calculating a percentage of compliance, it is not recommended that

the therapist use fewer than 10 occurrences. This recommendation may help the therapist determine the interval to use when reporting data. For instance, if more than 10 opportunities for measurement occur each day, then it is reasonable to calculate and share the compliance data on a daily basis. The reason for recommending a minimum of 10 occurrences is that if fewer than 10 are used, it is often difficult to recognize subtle trends in the client's performance. Although this approach is not statistically rigorous, I have found that it works well in clinical use. In general, the accuracy of the compliance data improves as more occurrences are used. Situations in which conclusions are based on only 2 or 3 occurrences should be avoided.

Charting the client's percentage of compliance over time provides a means of visualizing the client's long-term progress. The trends discovered by plotting the client's percentage of compliance versus time often help define an emphasis for continued treatment. Figure 3.4 shows an example chart summarizing the data gathered for a client's compliance in checking her

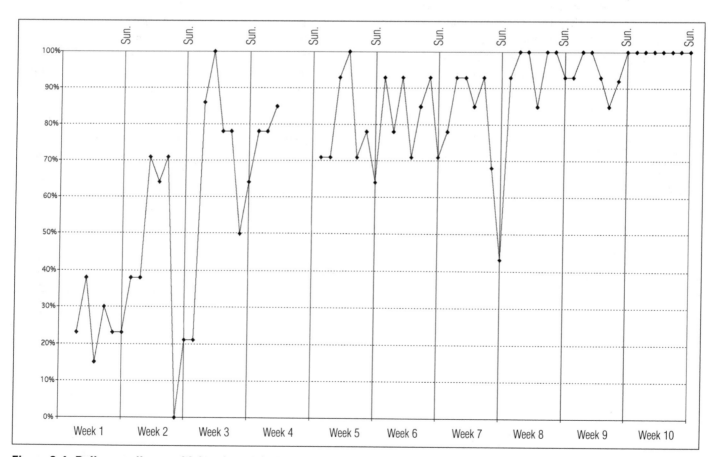

Figure 3.4. Daily compliance with hourly watch chime.
Note. Data are missing for Week 4.

organizer at the sound of her hourly watch chime. In this case the client had more than 10 opportunities per day, and a percentage of compliance was calculated daily. This example illustrates the nonlinear behavior typical of most clients' progress. Her percentage of compliance did not steadily rise from each day to the next. During the first 2 weeks, large declines in compliance were observed on weekends when her daily schedule was less structured. These weekend declines affected her performance on Mondays. She tended to have the most compliance mid-week when the routine of checking her organizer carried over from the previous weekday. By plotting and reviewing the data on a daily basis, it became clear in the first couple of weeks that the treatment plan needed to focus more on weekends. By the third week we began to focus more on weekends. The client's compliance steadily improved from there. After 9 weeks she reached 100% compliance in referring to her organizer when her watch chimed each hour. If this same data had instead been plotted on a weekly basis, then the daily fluctuation would not have been so clear. Eventually we might have realized that the weekends were a problem, but it probably would have taken more time to figure that out.

It should be noted that not all clients benefit from reviewing their compliance data. Although it is usually recommended that the data be shared with the client and family, situations will sometimes arise when such sharing is counterproductive. In some cases, especially if the client is just beginning to comprehend the severity of his or her deficits, pointing out the degree of noncompliance can be overwhelming. It is, of course, up to the therapist to determine what should be shared and when. Sharing the data is meant to support, not obstruct, the overall goals of the treatment plan.

Knowing When to Terminate Data Collection. It is not always apparent when to quit collecting compliance data. Making accurate measurements of a client's compliance is not an effortless process. It takes the continued commitment of members of the support network and a substantial amount of the therapist's time. Because of the effort involved, the data collection process cannot continue indefinitely. If the client has reached 100% compliance for a satisfactory time, there is no reason to keep measuring. In many cases, however, the client never reaches 100% compliance, and a different criterion for ceasing data collection will need to be determined.

There are two basic reasons for collecting data: (1) to document the client's progress and (2) to provide information that helps define the focus of the treatment plan. When data collection does not support either of these objectives, then it is probably time to stop gathering data. Do not be overly concerned about stopping the data collection too early because it is always possible to resume it later if needed. In many cases it is appropriate to stop collecting data once the client has achieved an acceptable level of compliance and then periodically gather additional data to monitor the client's ability to sustain that level of compliance.

Modification Phase

As the treatment plan is executed and measured, it will be apparent that certain techniques are working well and others are not. This usually becomes clear during the measurement phase, as the client's performance is monitored. The techniques that are working well should be emphasized, and those that are not should be modified, stopped, and tried again later or eliminated from the treatment plan. Sometimes it is not only the techniques that need to be modified; the measurement data may show that the stated goal is unreachable and needs to be adjusted.

It is not recommended that a distinct time in the treatment plan be set up to make all changes. Modifications should be made throughout the treatment process whenever warranted. The therapist is cautioned to give the initial treatment plan or previous modifications time to work before making changes. Continue with the current process until a clear trend, based on measurement data, support network feedback, or direct observations, is established.

Summary

The development of an effective memory compensation system is a learning process that requires frequent review and modification as it evolves toward success. The implementation cycle in Figure 3.1 will be repeated numerous times during the treatment of any given client. Among other things, the goals of treatment will be revised, the roles of the members of the support network will change, and various memory compensation tools will be added or deleted. However, the basic cycle of planning, executing, measuring, and modifying will continue as long as the client remains in therapy.

Case Examples Using a Memory Compensation System

The five cases that follow are intended to provide functional examples of the use of the memory compensation tools described in this book. I selected these cases because I feel that they represent the range of clients that most therapists will encounter.

The first case (Case A) describes my work with a client who was very confused and had little or no awareness of his environment. As might be expected, this client had severe memory and cognitive deficits. I have included this example because it describes how I began treatment with a client with very-low-level functioning and how I modified the approach as the client improved.

The second case (Case B) describes my work with a client with a severe memory deficit. Treatment was concentrated on teaching her to carry her personal organizer with her, to make entries in the organizer, and to refer to it often. The goal was to establish a foundation on which she could build when she transitioned from the hospital into a residential treatment program.

The client in the third case (Case C) had physical, speech, and language deficits, as well as memory impairment. Organizer use is often overlooked for clients with this combination of problems. Various techniques that I used to help her compensate for her deficits are described.

The fourth case (Case D) describes a client whose primary goal was to become independent with home management. She was experiencing problems structuring and initiating her activities of daily living (ADL). The treatment strategy centered around use of a personal organizer, forms, and checklists.

The last case (Case E) describes a client with moderate memory deficits who was attempting to run a small business. He was relatively high-level functioning. His case is included because it shows the use of an elaborate organizer system using all components.

Case Example A: Inpatient Rehabilitation

27-Year-Old Man With a Right Frontal Parietal Brain Injury Caused by a Fall

Illustrated in this example:
- Treatment strategy for a confused client with severe cognitive deficits (passive client)
- Use of basic orientation materials
- Structuring the environment
- Progression to a modified memory notebook
- Team treatment approach
- Benefits of a strong support network

Initial Evaluation

This client was admitted to the hospital following a fall. The initial evaluation took place (on the rehabilitation unit) 2 weeks after his injury. The client was severely confused and oriented only to self. He required constant cuing to complete basic tasks, such as dressing, grooming, and showering. Without cuing he would not initiate such tasks or would be distracted before completing them.

He had a semiprivate room on the rehabilitation unit and would often mistakenly use his roommate's belongings. He was unable to locate his room within the rehabilitation unit, and when in his room he could not remember which bed was his. He would often be found lying in his roommate's bed.

Focus of Treatment

I considered this client "passive," meaning that he had no awareness or insight into his situation and thus was not actively attempting to compensate for his problems. With this type of client, the therapist needs to provide a highly structured environment that will allow the client to function at a basic level. The initial focus of treatment should be on basic orientation.

Developing Basic Orientation Materials

The client could consistently remember his name and identify family members but was unable to remember either where he was or what the date was each day. My goal for the orientation of this client was for him to be able to consistently recall those items.

I have witnessed therapists working with similar clients who each day will ask the client basic orientation questions (e.g., Where are you? What month/year is it?), and each time the client guesses and answers incorrectly. The therapist then corrects the client and moves on. Five minutes later when asked the same questions, the client again guesses and answers incorrectly. I believe that this method of treatment does very little to improve the basic orientation of the client.

My approach is to provide the client with reference material and then teach the client to access it. In this case I used the dry-erase board in the client's room to post a clearly visible sign that read, "St. Joseph's Hospital, Phoenix, Arizona." Beneath that I wrote the month, day, and year. I conducted my therapy sessions in the client's room, and sometimes as many as 20 times each session I would ask the client the basic orientation questions. Before he could guess at an answer, I would direct his attention to the dry-erase board. My intention was to teach him to reference the board before answering the questions. Of course, the client's responses were only as accurate as the posted information. Therefore, I set up a system using nursing staff and family members to ensure that the day and date information was always updated. Gradually the client learned to automatically reference the posted signs when asked basic orientation questions.

At first glance it may seem unproductive to teach the client to automatically reference a posted sign. After all, when he leaves the hospital he will not be able to reference that sign. My reason for doing this is simple: It teaches him to use reference materials rather than guessing to answer questions. It also prepares him for using more complex compensations, such as notebooks and personal organizers, as his condition improves. All of us use a similar technique every day when we need to know the time of day. We instinctively look at a watch or a clock because we know it will be more accurate than guessing.

Structuring the Environment

An approach consisting of signs and labels similar to that used for basic orientation was used to provide a well-defined, structured environment for the client. As observed during the initial evaluation, this client was unable to locate his room or remember which bed was his. I started by posting signs with his name on the outside of the door to his room, on the wall above his bed, and on the door to his closet. His personal hygiene items (e.g., toothbrush, razor) also were labeled and placed in a container with his name on it. His side of the bathroom counter was labeled so that he could keep his items separate from his roommate's.

An important aspect of structuring the environment is keeping it organized over time. For example, the client might pick up his comb from the bathroom to comb his hair and then leave it next to his bed. At the beginning of each therapy session, I would work with the client to return all misplaced items to their designated place. Then during the session if an item such as the comb was used, I would cue the client to return it to its designated place immediately. I also instructed all of the members of the client's support network to do the same.

Defining a Routine

At the time of initial treatment, the client was so confused and easily distracted that he was unable to complete even a simple series of tasks, such as those associated with a morning routine. For instance, he might remember to shave but forget to brush his teeth, take a shower, or put on clean clothes. Even if I told him specifically to take a shower, he might be distracted and forget to do it.

The client needed a well-defined procedure to follow to complete these tasks. I generated the checklist shown in Figure 4.1 for him to follow. The checklist was written on a placard and posted on the wall where he would easily see it. I scheduled my therapy sessions early each morning right after he had finished breakfast. The first task on the checklist was "eat breakfast." The

---

Morning Routine

☐ Eat breakfast

☐ Go to closet and pick out clean clothes

☐ Shower

☐ Dress

☐ Brush teeth

☐ Shave

☐ Comb hair

Figure 4.1. Morning checklist, as used in Case A.

client was instructed to place a check in the box next to that task and then continue on to the next task until all tasks were completed. I arranged to have two sessions each day with this client. During the afternoon session I would erase the check marks from the completed checklist to prepare it for the next morning.

The purpose of using this simple checklist was twofold. First, it prompted the client to complete the needed tasks, and it also provided training to get him to reference external cues. I anticipated that this client would progress and continue to use checklists and other external cues as he needed to learn new procedures and information. The expectation was that at some point he would develop a routine and no longer need to reference this checklist to perform his morning tasks. Similar checklists could be used to teach him different routines as appropriate.

Evolution of Treatment

After about 2 weeks of following the basic procedures discussed above, the client began to show a marked improvement. He progressed to the point that he no longer needed to use the checklist to complete his morning tasks. He was less distractible and was able to provide basic orientation information without always

having to reference the posted signs. I was able to remove most of the labels on his personal items (e.g., toothbrush, razor, closet, bed). Now that he was comfortable with his environment within his room, it was time to start increasing the complexity of the tasks that he would be expected to complete.

At this point I felt that the client was ready to begin using a basic memory notebook, a brightly colored folder or 3-ring binder that the client would take with him throughout the day. I labeled the front of the notebook with the client's name and room number. Inside the notebook I set up sections that included
• A monthly calendar (Figure 4.2),
• A brief medical history (Figure 4.3),
• The client's therapy schedule (Figure 4.4),
• A map of the rehabilitation unit and written directions to and from therapy sessions (Figure 4.5), and
• Staff names and photographs.

It was important not to make the notebook too complicated and thus risk confusing the client. The monthly calendar was included solely to help the client remember the day and date. He did not keep any notes or plan future events with this calendar. I instructed other staff to always check his calendar to make sure that all past days were crossed off.

Month: *February*						Year: *2005*
Sunday	**Monday**	**Tuesday**	**Wednesday**	**Thursday**	**Friday**	**Saturday**
		1	*2*	*3*	*4*	*5*
6	*7*	*8*	*9*	*10*	*11*	*12*
13	*14*	*15*	*16*	*17*	*18*	*19*
20	*21*	*22*	*23*	*24*	*25*	*26*
27	*28*					

Figure 4.2. Monthly calendar, as used in Case A.

- Admitted to St. Joseph's Hospital, Phoenix, Arizona, on January 21, 2001.

- Fell off a roof while working.

- Suffered a brain injury.

Figure 4.3. Brief medical history, as used in Case A.

The medical history section provided a brief summary of the client's hospital course that he could reference at any time. He might use it if asked questions about why he was in the hospital or how long it had been since his accident. He also would review it frequently throughout each day so that he could become more familiar with the circumstances regarding his hospitalization.

A weekly therapy schedule listing all sessions and activities also was included. At the end of each session the therapist was instructed to cue the client to cross

Time	Monday	Tuesday	Wednesday	Thursday	Friday	Saturday	Sunday
7:00 AM							
8:00 AM	Occupational Therapy	Occupational Therapy	Occupational Therapy	Occupational Therapy	Occupational Therapy		
9:00 AM			Physical Therapy			Occupational Therapy	
10:00 AM	Physical Therapy	Physical Therapy		Physical Therapy	Physical Therapy		
11:00 AM	Speech Therapy	Speech Therapy	Speech Therapy	Speech Therapy	Speech Therapy	Physical Therapy/Speech Therapy	
12:00 NOON			Cooking Group			Group Outing	
1:00 PM	Physical Therapy	Physical Therapy	Physical Therapy	Physical Therapy	Physical Therapy		
2:00 PM	Speech Therapy	Speech Therapy	Speech Therapy	Speech Therapy	Speech Therapy	Speech Therapy	
3:00 PM	Occupational Therapy	Occupational Therapy	Occupational Therapy	Occupational Therapy	Occupational Therapy		
4:00 PM		Group Outing					
5:00 PM							

Figure 4.4. Therapy schedule, as used in Case A.

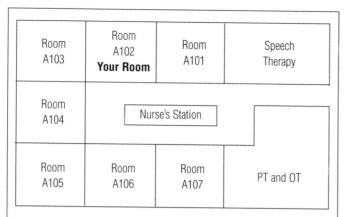

Room A103	Room A102 **Your Room**	Room A101	Speech Therapy
Room A104	Nurse's Station		
Room A105	Room A106	Room A107	PT and OT

DIRECTIONS TO THERAPY

To Speech Therapy:
- Go left out of your room to the end of the hall.
- Find office door marked "Dennis."

To Physical Therapy and Occupational Therapy:
- Go left out of your room and go right around the end of the Nurse's Station.
- Find door marked "PT/OT Gym."

DIRECTIONS TO YOUR ROOM FROM THERAPY

From Speech Therapy:
- Exit Dennis's office and go right.
- Follow hall to Room A102 (on your right).

From Physical Therapy and Occupational Therapy:
- Exit the PT/OT Gym.
- Go straight toward Nurse's Station.
- Turn left after Nurse's Station.
- Follow hall to Room A102 (on your right).

Figure 4.5. Map of rehabilitation unit and written directions to therapy sessions, as used in Case A.

that session off his schedule. In addition, each therapist was responsible for reviewing the client's therapy schedule and making any updates if the scheduled time for any upcoming sessions needed to be changed.

Because this client had great difficulty learning his way around the rehabilitation unit, detailed directions to the location of each therapy session were included in his notebook. As illustrated in Figure 4.5, a map of the unit indicating his room and landmarks within the unit, such as the nurse's station, was provided. Written directions from his room to each session, as well as directions back to his room, also were included.

The final section of the client's notebook included the names and photographs of staff members involved in his direct care.

The focus of my treatment turned to teaching the client to use his basic memory notebook. My approach was to provide him with many opportunities each day to reference the notebook so that he would develop a routine of referring to it when necessary. The first step was to make sure that the notebook was available at all times. A specific place on his bed stand was designated for his notebook. A sign, such as in Figure 4.6, was placed above his bed directing the staff to make sure that he would take his notebook when he left his room.

During my therapy sessions I would ask the client specific questions about the information in his notebook. For instance, I might ask him what time he had physical therapy that day. He was expected to immediately reference his notebook. If he did not, I would cue him to do so and help him access the proper information. I instructed other staff to do the same.

Over the next 2 weeks, the client became more and more independent with using his notebook. He was able to get to therapy sessions independently approximately 70 percent of the time. At that point the client was discharged to an outpatient therapy program.

Summary

This client was in the beginning stages of recovery from his brain injury, and it was unclear what his long-term prognosis would be. Because I had only 4 weeks to work with him, I focused primarily on defining a foundation on which he could build as he improved. The client was at a stage at which all of the compensations had to be kept at a very basic level. Providing a structure to his environment that would help him cope with his confusion was of primary importance.

Another aspect of this case that cannot be overstated is that the client needed a consistent treatment approach with much repetition to improve. Many times the therapist gets bored with going through the "same

John Doe has a memory notebook.

Description: Red 3-ring binder.

Location: Stored in the red plastic bin on his bedside table.

Please remind him to take it with him when he leaves the room.

Figure 4.6. Notebook reminder sign, as used in Case A.

old routine" each day and seeks ways to add variety to the therapy sessions. In this case, with a highly confused client, adding variety would have been counterproductive. The client needed the opportunity to master basic skills before moving on.

Case Example B: Inpatient Rehabilitation

38-Year-Old Married Woman With 3 Children With Subarachnoid Bleed From Aneurysm in Left Posterior Cerebellar Artery

Illustrated in this example:

- Treatment strategy for a client with dense amnesia
- Selection of an appropriate personal organizer
- Using a watch in conjunction with daily organizer pages
- Organizer use to decrease confabulation
- Team treatment approach
- Benefits of a strong support network

Initial Evaluation

This client was first evaluated 14 weeks after having a subarachnoid bleed from an aneurysm in the left posterior cerebellar artery. During the 14 weeks before my evaluation, she had received acute rehabilitation in the hospital and was transferred to a residential rehabilitation program, but then she was readmitted to the acute rehabilitation unit following a grand mal seizure. When I began working with her, she required close medical monitoring and was expected to stay in acute rehabilitation for another 4 weeks, after which she would return to the residential program.

During my initial evaluation of the client, she demonstrated dense amnesia. She was not oriented to place or time, could not find her room, could not recall having visitors, and could not remember what she had recently eaten. When asked questions, such as what she had done the previous day, she tended to confabulate responses rather than admitting that she could not remember. Results of the Rivermead Behavioural Memory Test (Wilson et al., 1989) indicated severe memory impairment.

Focus of Treatment

That this client was more than 3 months' post–brain injury and continued to display a dense amnesic syndrome indicated that her memory impairment was unlikely to improve anytime soon. If her memory did not significantly improve, she would eventually need a comprehensive memory compensation system to reach a basic level of functional independence. During my 4 weeks with the client, my plan was to provide a solid foundation for continued expansion of the use of memory compensation tools after she left my facility. Participation of her family would be a key element, not only during my 4 weeks of treatment but also to provide continuity of the approach once she returned to the residential program.

Selecting the Personal Organizer

The first order of business was to select an appropriate personal organizer. The client's high degree of memory impairment meant that she would need to track a large amount of information in her organizer. She had good reading and writing skills and no major physical problems. She also had a very supportive family that was willing to participate in the treatment plan. All of these traits made her an excellent candidate for a comprehensive system, including all elements of an organizer. However, in the 4 weeks I had to work with her, I knew that we would be able to focus only on the use of a watch with an alarm in conjunction with the daily pages. A full-sized (8 ½ x 11 inch) organizer was purchased. The sections, including the month-in-a-view calendars, to-do lists, and other items, were removed but not discarded because they would eventually be needed. Only the predated daily pages remained. A wristwatch with an hourly chime and alarm also was purchased. I gave her instructions for using the watch (refer to Chapter 3, Figure 3.2) and created a section in the organizer in which to keep them.

Defining the Roles of the Support Network

On the rehabilitation unit the client interacted with nursing staff, other therapists, and physicians. In addition, members of her family were with her each evening and on weekends. The initial goal of treatment was to teach her to refer to her organizer each hour during the day when her watch chimed. To accomplish this she needed to keep her watch and organizer with her at all times. Because no single person was with her throughout the day, the coordinated assistance of her support network was crucial to achieve this goal. I met with the nursing staff, other therapists, her physician, and family and communicated my treatment plan. All of them agreed that, if she left her room without her watch and organizer, they would accompany her back to her room to retrieve them. This applied even when she took short trips to the nursing station or went outside to smoke a cigarette. This helped her develop a habit of always taking her organizer no matter where she went.

The other responsibility of the support network was to make sure that the client always opened her organizer and made an entry immediately after the watch chimed each hour. They were instructed to cue her to do so if she did not initiate this task immediately. We also made arrangements to ensure that there was always someone with her each hour throughout the day between 8:00 a.m. and 8:00 p.m. when the watch chimed.

Making Entries

I instructed the client to make hourly entries consisting of a short note describing what she was doing at the time. My intent was to provide her with many opportunities to make entries so that she would learn to refer to her organizer often and also to give her a written history of her day to augment her memory. She had good language skills and was able to write legibly but had difficulty writing meaningful, concise notes and placing them in the correct location on the daily pages. When her watch chimed I instructed her to check the time and date on her watch and find the corresponding location on the daily pages to make the entry. She was impulsive, and if she did not develop the habit of checking her watch first, she would frequently make entries in the wrong location. After she found the correct location, I told her to write down what she was doing. At first she had difficulty wording the notes, so I would dictate them to her (e.g., eating lunch, watching TV news). The other members of her support network were trained to follow this same procedure. After about 3 weeks she was able to compose her own notes but still required verbal cuing to ensure that she made the entries.

In addition to the hourly entries, I began working with the client on using her organizer to complete assignments. This was particularly important because her severe memory impairment kept her from performing all but the most routine tasks. The entries for assignments differed from the hourly entries in two ways. First, each entry contained a note for which an action needed to be performed. Second, the entries were made anytime the assignment was given, not just on the hour. Because the hourly entries were recorded next to each hourly time slot, the assignments had to be recorded in a different location on the daily pages as shown in Figure 4.7.

An important aspect of the assignments was that they had to be verifiable. The client had a tendency to confabulate, so I gave only assignments that I could verify. For example, one of her assignments was to record what she ate for meals each day. I met with her dietitian and obtained daily copies of her menu. I could then verify the accuracy of her entries. Other example assign-

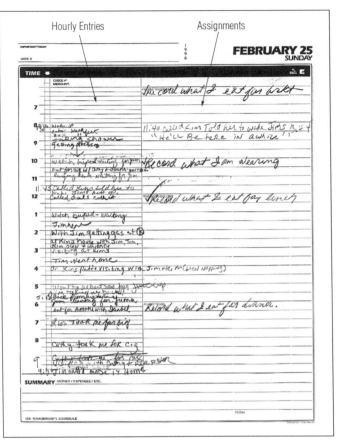

Figure 4.7. Example daily page with hourly entries and assignments, as used in Case B.

ments included recording what she wore each day, and placing phone calls to my answering machine, which would record not only the instructed message but also the time of day the call was placed.

I set up a separate section in her organizer where simple forms, as shown in Figure 4.8, were placed for her to record what she ate and what she wore each day. These forms provided an organized location for her to enter the information from her assignments. Without the forms, she tended to make entries out of sequence in various places throughout her organizer. This made it nearly impossible for her to later reference the information. As with the hourly notes, she initially required assistance with recording the information in the correct section and location on the form. It took her about 3 weeks to independently initiate making these entries.

Retrieving Information

The first step to begin working on retrieving information was to teach the client to immediately refer to her organizer whenever her watch chimed or when asked a question. As usual, my approach was to provide many

DAY	BREAKFAST	LUNCH	DINNER
Sunday			
Monday			
Tuesday			
Wednesday			
Thursday			
Friday			
Saturday			

Figure 4.8. Example form for recording meals, as used in Case B. (Similar form was used for recording clothing.)

opportunities throughout the day for her to practice. I would ask her questions about the clothes she wore, what activities she participated in, what she ate at mealtime, and other items that I knew she had recorded in her organizer. She was expected to immediately reference her organizer for the answer. If she did not, I would cue her to do so and, if necessary, help her locate where the information was recorded. For example, when asked what she ate for breakfast, she was expected to open her organizer to the section titled "What I Ate," and look up the information. Because I was with her only about 3 hours each day, I trained the members of her support network to follow the same procedure.

Of course, it was impossible to record information about every question the client might be asked. This client's first inclination when she did not have recorded data was to confabulate. For example, she might be asked what she had watched on television. Even though she was not tracking that information, she would thumb through her organizer to see if she had the answer and, if not, she would make up a response. Even with the items she was tracking, she would sometimes forget to make an entry if not properly cued. If asked later what she wore on Wednesday she might find a blank in the "What I Wore" section for that day, and her inclination

was to confabulate. A major focus of my treatment was to teach her to admit that she could not remember when such a situation occurred. Rather than making up a response, I instructed her to say "I don't know. I don't have it written down." As usual, the members of her support network were instructed to follow the same procedure. It did not take her long to get in the habit of admitting that she could not remember things that were not written down.

Summary

Because I had only 4 weeks to work with this client, I was able to provide only a foundation for using memory compensation tools. When she left my care she was able to refer to the appropriate section of her organizer independently when information was requested about 75% of the time. She was consistently entering information, recording what she ate and wore in the appropriate sections. She also was able to verbally acknowledge her inability to remember information, instead of confabulating, approximately 95% of the time. These skills were the necessary first step in teaching her to use her organizer to help meet her daily needs.

After leaving my care this client returned to a residential program where she continued to receive daily therapies. To provide continuity of care I shared my treatment plan with her new therapists. Because I had worked closely with her family members, they also were able to help provide continuity. Although I have not been in direct contact with this client since she left my care, her physician has told me that she continues to make progress with organizer use even though she has had no significant memory improvement.

Case Example C: Outpatient Day Treatment Program

35-Year-Old Woman, Kindergarten Teacher With Subarachnoid Hemorrhage, Ruptured Left Ophthalmic Artery Aneurysm, and CVA Following Craniotomy

Illustrated in this example:
- Preliminary evaluation techniques to define appropriate memory compensation tools
- Use of customized instruction sheets
- Adaptations for a client with hemiplegia and speech and language deficits
- Evaluation and treatment in the client's environment
- Benefits of a strong support system

Initial Evaluation

This client entered an outpatient day treatment program after spending approximately 5 months in an acute care hospital and an inpatient rehabilitation facility. She had significant deficits in cognition, speech and language, visual perception, and right-side motor control. Her cognitive deficits included memory, speed of information processing, sequencing, and an overall decreased awareness of her situation. Her speech and language deficits included moderate aphasia (both expressive and receptive) and oral apraxia. She had difficulty naming, reading, writing to dictation, and copying. She was right-side dominant, and the hemiplegia affected that side, leaving her with no functional use of her right arm. She was ambulating with a straight cane for short distances and using a wheelchair in the community.

This client had strong family support. She was married and living at home with her husband and parents. Her parents were retired and had temporarily moved in with the client and her husband to help care for her.

During my initial evaluation of the client, it became clear that her inability to complete basic ADL created a considerable hardship for her family. If she could become independent with the following items, her family would be able to return to a fairly normal lifestyle:
• Bathing, dressing, grooming, and taking medications
• Doing laundry, cooking meals, and cleaning
• Being able to be left unsupervised for up to 10 hours.
In addition, the client indicated that she was unable to accurately recall and communicate details about her personal history. She had only a mild memory deficit, but the effects of aphasia made it seem more severe. She was frustrated and embarrassed when unable to communicate items such as her address, telephone number, medical history, and family relationships.

It seemed clear from the start that this client was motivated to improve her independence so that she would not be a burden on her family. Her husband and parents seemed very supportive, willing to follow the program of treatment, and realistic regarding the effort required of them. They also seemed to understand that the level of independence that she would likely achieve would be significantly less than she had before her brain injury. These factors made her a good candidate for an intensive therapy program.

Focus of Treatment

It was clear from the beginning that, because of her ADL deficiencies, this client would not be able to immediately start using a comprehensive memory compensation system. A treatment plan with initial emphasis on basic ADL and limited personal organizer use would be followed. As independence with ADL was achieved, more emphasis on

organizer use would be included. The long-term goal was independence within the home, not a return to work. To learn the details of the client's home life, numerous visits to the client's home would be necessary.

A treatment plan consisting of daily sessions with the client and weekly sessions with the family was set up. Most of the sessions took place in the clinic, but it was necessary to visit the home at least once a week. Traditional occupational therapy focusing on the client's physical impairments was included during the clinical sessions. The family not only participated during the home visits but also came to the clinic when requested.

Initial Short-Term Goals (Weeks 1–4)

During my initial sessions with the family, they reported several items that were causing frustration within their household. In particular, the client was unable to independently use the toilet at night, was unable to bathe or dress herself, and was not independent with taking her medications. She required intense supervision and assistance from her family members to complete any of these tasks. Independence with each of these items became the initial goals of therapy.

Using the Toilet at Night. The client required an ankle–foot orthosis to ambulate during the day. She required assistance to don the brace, and after removing the brace at night she used a wheelchair. Because she was unsafe with transfers from the wheelchair, she would wake up her husband to assist her in the bathroom at night.

My first step was to observe the client in her home performing this activity. It was immediately clear that her sequencing and memory deficits, not her physical impairments, were the root of the problem. She did not lock the brakes or place both feet on the floor before transferring from her wheelchair, and she grabbed unstable objects for support.

My approach was simple: Post brief instructions for transfers in a prominent place in the bathroom and train the client and family about their use. The instructions shown in Figure 4.9 were posted on a placard next to the toilet. Each night the client's husband would place her wheelchair by her bed with the brakes locked. Initially, her husband continued to accompany her to the toilet, but instead of physically assisting her with the transfer, he would cue her to refer to the posted instructions to ensure that she followed each step. Within 2 weeks she was performing transfers correctly without cuing, and her husband could sleep through the night.

Although it is not immediately obvious, training the client for safe transfers was a beginning step toward

---

TO USE TOILET

1. Lock both wheelchair brakes.

2. Put both feet on floor.

3. Reach for toilet arm.

    DO NOT USE TOWEL RACK!

Figure 4.9. Instructions for toilet transfers, as used in Case C.

organizer use. The process required her to access written information and precisely follow a defined procedure, the same steps she would later follow when using an organizer.

Bathing and Dressing. As with the use of the toilet, through initial observations it was apparent that the client's sequencing and memory deficits, not physical impairments, were preventing her from being independent with bathing and dressing. A similar approach relying on brief but detailed instruction sheets was followed. An example of her "after-shower" instruction sheet is shown in Figure 4.10. These instructions were posted on a placard in the bathroom where she would see them each day. Similar placards were placed inside her shower and in her bedroom, where she dressed each

---

AFTER SHOWER

1. Towel off.

2. Put lotion on face.

3. Put lotion on legs.

4. Use deodorant.

5. Mousse hair.

6. Comb hair.

7. Blow dry hair.

8. Use hairspray.

9. Apply make-up.

10. Put powder on feet.

11. Dress.

12. Eat breakfast.

13. Brush teeth.

14. Use toilet.

Figure 4.10. Example of "after-shower" instruction sheet, as used in Case C.

day. Her husband and parents initially cued her to complete each item in the proper order, and after about 2 weeks she was independent with bathing and dressing.

Taking Medications. The client needed to take several different pills 3 times per day. Realizing that she was not reliable with this task, her family assumed the responsibility. My approach for making her independent with this task was to use an organizer in conjunction with a weekly pillbox. I recommended to her husband that he purchase a medium-sized personal organizer with daily dated pages and a pillbox with three dosing compartments for each day of the week. Each week the family would place the medications in her pillbox. I worked with the client to teach her to write a simple note in her organizer each day at 7:00 a.m., noon, and 6:00 p.m. to remind her to take her medications. During therapy sessions I reviewed her organizer and ensured that the word *medication* was written at the proper time slots for the next week. If there were problems, I helped her make the necessary corrections.

Rather than using a watch alarm to remind her to check her organizer, the medications were coordinated with mealtimes. At each meal she was cued by a family member or therapist to reference her organizer. Immediately after taking the medications (and only after, not before), she would place a check mark next to the entry in her organizer. After the first couple of days she routinely checked her organizer at each meal and several other times throughout the day. This client did not need any assistance in learning to keep her organizer with her at all times.

The pillbox provided a means of verifying that the medications had indeed been taken. Sometimes she would take the medications but forget to place a check mark in her organizer. Other times she would not take the medications at all. By the end of Week 4 she still required cuing about 30% of the time for this task.

Revised Short-Term Goals (Weeks 5–8)

At this point in the treatment the client was able to independently follow the instruction sheets for bathing, dressing, and using the toilet, but she still required direct assistance with her medications. While continuing to work on the medications, new goals involving basic home tasks and unsupervised time were pursued. Please note that I make no distinction between the term *instruction sheets* that I have been using in this example and the term *procedures* as described in Chapter 2.

Taking Medications. Because the client did not meet the goal of 100% independence with taking her medications during the first 4 weeks of treatment, this continued to be a focus of treatment. We continued to follow the same procedure described earlier, with a couple of modifications. Rather than immediately cuing the client at the defined time, she was given approximately 10 minutes to remember to take her medications. If she still forgot, then she would be cued by a family member or therapist. The other change involved the use of a rubber stamp to make the entries in her organizer. Her speech and language deficits made it difficult for her to accurately write entries on the daily pages. A rubber stamp with the word "medications" was used to make it easier for her. By the end of the 8th week she was independent with this task.

Performing Home Tasks. The client had a strong desire to assist with basic home chores such as doing laundry, using a microwave oven, and cleaning the bathroom. As with the previous ADL, her memory and sequencing deficits, not her physical impairments, were the major problem. My approach was to once again construct detailed instruction sheets (i.e., procedures) for each task. During my weekly sessions in her home, we spent a substantial amount of time going through and recording the steps of each task. Instruction sheets for using the washer and dryer were posted on a placard in the laundry room. An instruction sheet for cleaning the bathroom was posted in her bathroom. Numerous recipes were adapted and placed in a folder in her kitchen.

The importance of developing the instruction sheet in the environment where the task will be performed cannot be overstated. By observing the client and making modifications to the instruction sheets as she performed each task, I was able to see the client's shortcomings and provide instructions to overcome them. For example, a certain recipe shown in Figure 4.11 required cooking in the microwave oven for 12 minutes. The client, however, would repeatedly enter 12 seconds. Upon observing this, I modified the recipe to indicate 12:00 minutes in the same format as shown on the oven timer for the cooking time. This small change made her independent with the activity.

By the end of the 8th week the client required only occasional assistance with doing laundry, following simple recipes, and cleaning the bathroom.

Having Unsupervised Time. The client's parents planned on returning to their own home once their daughter was able to care for herself. The client's husband also planned on returning to work and leaving her alone at home during the day. Our primary concern was that her language and mobility deficits would prevent her from summoning assistance if some emergency occurred during the day.

PIZZA

1. Check oven—Place rack on center shelf.
2. Preheat oven to 450 degrees.
3. When oven light goes off, oven is ready.
4. Take pizza out of plastic bag.
5. Put pizza on a cookie sheet.
6. Place on center rack in oven—USE HOTPADS!
7. Bake for 12:00 minutes—SET TIMER.
8. Remove from oven—USE HOTPADS!
9. TURN OFF OVEN.
10. Cut pizza and serve.

Figure 4.11. Modified recipe, as used in Case C.

My first recommendation was that the family arrange for a personal response system to be installed at the house. Such a system would allow the client to summon assistance by simply pressing a button on a bracelet or necklace that she would wear at all times. An important feature was that the client would have to actively reset the system at predefined intervals each day. If the system was not reset, the monitoring center would assume that the client needed help and call for assistance. To use the system the client would have to remember to reset it twice each day. Entries were made in her organizer to remind her to reset the system. As with the medications, a rubber stamp was used to make the entries.

We started with 1 hour of unsupervised time per day several times a week and gradually increased the time. This worked well and, within a couple of months, the client was frequently left home alone for up to 10 hours with no problems.

By the end of the 8th week the client was independently using her organizer to track medications and reset the personal response system. The client and her family also began to find the organizer useful for entering other information such as appointments, weekend plans, and reminder notes. Because of her speech and language problems, the family often made the entries for her. Writing her own entries soon became one of her primary goals.

Revised Short-Term Goals (Weeks 9–12)

By this point the client was independent with her medications. She also was able to complete simple home tasks with only minor assistance and was making progress on unsupervised time at home. With these items under control, the focus of treatment shifted to personal organizer use. The goal for the next 4 weeks was for the client to take increased responsibility for making entries and retrieving information from her organizer.

Making Entries in the Organizer. As mentioned earlier, the client was using rubber stamps to make entries for medications and resetting the personal response system. Most other entries, such as appointments and "to-do" items, were made by her family and me. She had been working with a speech therapist on writing to dictation and spelling and had reached a point at which she was beginning to formulate and write simple notes. Now she was ready to start focusing on the mechanics of organizer use.

To use her organizer independently, the client needed to be able to formulate meaningful notes and record them in the proper place. During therapy sessions I concentrated on providing the client with many opportunities to practice. I gave her assignments that included an action that needed to be performed by her at a specific time, such as making a telephone call or bringing a particular item to the next session. Each assignment provided an occasion for her to practice finding the correct location in her organizer to make a meaningful entry. By observing her approach to the assignments, I was able to determine her shortcomings.

This client was quickly able to understand the structure of her organizer and find the proper locations for entries. However, due to spelling problems associated with aphasia, she had difficulty writing notes that she could understand and that captured the entire intent of the task. It was apparent that she could not independently overcome these deficits related to aphasia. She would need the help of others to make complete entries in her organizer.

My approach was to concentrate on teaching the client to request assistance when making entries in her organizer. She knew from her early success with using her organizer to help with medications and resetting her personal response system that use of an organizer could be of great benefit to her. Thus, she was eager to try this approach, even though it meant that she would constantly have to ask for the help of others, because she knew that, without their help, her language deficits would prevent her from effectively using her organizer.

We adopted a procedure for which each time she was given information to record, she would review her entry with the person who gave her the information. Everyone in her support network—family and other therapists—participated by cuing her to ask for help if

she did not request it. This approach worked well, and within 3 weeks the entries in her organizer were consistently accurate and complete. Although not technically independent with this aspect of organizer use, she took primary responsibility for making all entries and achieved a level of functionality that she could not have reached otherwise.

Retrieving Information

Usually the greatest barrier for retrieving information is remembering to refer to the organizer often. This client, however, had started using her organizer for medications during the first 4 weeks of treatment. By Week 9 she had acquired lots of practice and did not need reminders from her support network to reference her organizer. She also had little difficulty interpreting the entries that she had made if they were properly written. Nonetheless, her memory deficits in conjunction with the aphasia made it difficult for her to recall and communicate information. When asked for personal information, such as her birthdate, her memory problems might keep her from remembering it and, even if she did remember it, her aphasia might cause her to say the date incorrectly. If, however, the information was recorded in an accessible place, she could readily refer to it and read it back correctly when asked.

My approach was to define specific sections in her organizer containing needed personal information. Items including her address, phone number, medical history, names and birthdays of family members, educational history, and the like were listed in a personal history section of her organizer. This section was placed directly behind her daily pages, and a colored tab was used to make it easy to locate quickly. Her family members assumed the responsibility of adding or updating the information as needed. She rapidly became familiar with the items in that section and by Week 12 was independent with its use.

When I started working with this client it was clear that personal organizer use would have to be introduced very slowly. Her speech and language deficits could easily have prevented her from using an organizer at all. The early use of ADL instruction sheets provided the opportunity for the client and her family to recognize her potential for increased independence. It also provided a foundation for organizer use by teaching her to follow specific procedures. Once we saw how beneficial the ADL instruction sheets were, it was apparent that she was capable of using a more comprehensive system.

Many years after discharge from therapy, this client continues to use her organizer. She now lives independently with her husband and two children born since her brain injury. Through continued use of instruction sheets, she is able to care for her children during the day while her husband is at work. Throughout the years, additional organizer sections have been added for grocery shopping, child care, and even volunteer work.

Case Example D: Outpatient Rehabilitation

55-Year-Old Woman, Office Worker/Homemaker, 6 Months' Post-Resection of a Meningioma and 2 Years' Post-Surgical Clipping of a Left Ophthalmic Artery Aneurysm

Illustrated in this example:
- Development of compensations for home management activities
- Migration from simple to complex compensatory strategies

Initial Evaluation

This client had a complicated medical history; she was first evaluated 6 months after the resection of a right parafalcine meningioma and subsequent radiation therapy. One-and-a-half years before that, she had experienced aphasia and a right hemiparesis resulting from a left frontal intraparenchymal hemorrhage experienced during surgery to clip a left ophthalmic artery aneurysm. By the time I began working with her, she had made a good recovery from the aphasia and hemiparesis but was concerned about her failure to improve in her cognitive functioning. Results of her neuropsychological testing revealed a reduced capacity for verbal problem solving, nonverbal recall, and visuospatial problem solving. Difficulties with memory also were noted. In addition, she was on medication for depression.

The client arrived for her initial appointment with a spiral-bound notebook that she had purchased in an attempt to organize her daily activities. She also reported using a wall calendar at home to schedule appointments and a pillbox to ensure that her medications were taken. She told me that she had been very organized before her surgeries and had worked as a bookkeeper in her husband's business.

The client lived at home with her husband and 14-year-old daughter. She also had four other adult children who lived nearby. She came from a cultural background that placed a high degree of importance on having the wife/mother take care of all of the domestic duties around the house. This included meal planning and preparation, laundry, housekeeping, and child care. Her ability to complete these duties was a strong source

of pride to her before her surgeries, but since then she had experienced failures in all of them. She told me that she often made mistakes with bill paying and accumulated lots of late fees. She often would miss appointments and frequently forgot to pick up her daughter from after-school activities. She often was unable to think of anything to make for dinner, and when she did think of something she would never have it ready on time. At the grocery store she would buy items that were not needed and eventually have to throw them out when they spoiled. She became quite tearful during the evaluation, stating that her husband and daughter were frustrated with her inability to fulfill her responsibilities around the home. In fact, her daughter had begun seeing a counselor each week to help her adjust to the difficulties that her mother was experiencing.

The following deficits were apparent during the initial evaluation:
- Reduced mental stamina
- Decreased speed of information processing
- Memory impairment
- Organizational difficulties
- Decreased initiation.

These deficits were consistent with the client's medical history and neuropsychological test results. This client was a good candidate for treatment because of her awareness of her deficits and the effects that they were having on her day-to-day functioning. She had a strong motivation to improve her independence at home, and it was clear to me that she would work very hard to do so.

Focus of Treatment

From my initial contact with the client it was clear that she had no immediate desire to return to work. The entire focus of the treatment would be on teaching her to run her household effectively despite her deficits. I recommended that she purchase a medium-sized personal organizer with daily dated pages. It was clear that she would need checklists and forms to assist with activities such as bill paying, household chores, meal planning, and grocery shopping. But I did not feel that she would require the use of a watch with a chime/alarm, at least not initially.

I arranged to meet with the client twice per week for 3 months. Although most of the sessions would be at my office, a few sessions at her home would be necessary to see how her kitchen and home office were organized.

Initial Short-Term Goals (Weeks 1–4)

At the time that I began working with this client she was extremely frustrated by the impact that her deficits were having on her daily life. She had many items that she wanted to work on right away. However, I knew that if we tried to work on too many things at once, we would fail. Therefore, my approach was to select just a few items to work on initially. We worked together to select the following three items:

- Getting to appointments on time, including picking up her daughter from after-school activities
- Tracking medical information, including details of office visits with her doctors
- Independently doing the laundry each week

I felt that it was too early to begin working on more complex tasks such as meal planning and bill paying. An initial focus on the items above would allow us to concentrate on the basics of using memory compensation tools and to begin building a foundation for more complicated activities.

Keeping Appointments. When she first came to me, the client was recording appointments in a couple of places. The primary place was a wall calendar in her home where she recorded most of her appointments. She also had a spiral-bound notebook in which she would sometimes make notes. She had no routine established for checking either the wall calendar or notebook, so she often completely forgot about an upcoming appointment.

I began working with her on using her newly purchased personal organizer as the single location in which she would record all appointments. She had no problems keeping the organizer with her at all times, understanding its structure, and checking it frequently, but she did have difficulty making entries for new appointments. One common problem was that she would not enter the information for a new appointment immediately on receiving it. For example, if given a reminder card from her physician for her next appointment, she would often put the card in her purse and forget all about it. Similarly, if her daughter asked her for a ride home from school at a certain time, she would not immediately write it down and would soon become confused about what time to meet her daughter. Many times she would end up forgetting about it all together.

The first step was to get her to immediately make entries in her personal organizer when given the information. In this case the approach was very straightforward. I simply told the client that whenever she was given information about a new appointment, she was to enter it immediately in her organizer. If given a reminder card from a physician for an upcoming appointment, I instructed her to write the information in her organizer and throw the card away before leaving the office.

During subsequent treatment sessions for the next few weeks, I asked the client to go through her purse and look for any appointment reminder cards. Initially we found at least one or two that had not been entered in the organizer. I would instruct her to enter the information in her organizer and throw away the card.

At the client's request, her 14-year-old daughter was invited to attend a session for the purpose of educating her about her mother's memory deficits and the tools that she was using to compensate for them. I arranged with her daughter that every Sunday evening they would sit together and make entries in the organizer for all activities in the coming week. During the treatment sessions I would review her organizer pages to make sure that her daughter's activities were listed for the week. If I did not see the usual entries, I would have her make a note to review her organizer with her daughter that evening. After a while her daughter began writing short phrases of encouragement in her mother's organizer each day. Coming across a note like "Way to go, Mom" or "Thanks for picking me up" was very motivating for the client. Within 3 to 4 weeks she reduced her missed appointments to zero.

Managing Medical Information. Due to her complex medical history, the client was being seen by a variety of physicians. She required monthly lab work as well. To keep track of all of this, we included a medical information section in her organizer consisting of

- A clear plastic business card organizer in which we put a card from each of her medical providers (business card organizers such as this are usually available at office supply stores where personal organizers are sold);
- A form listing all of her medications, their purpose, and the prescribed dosage;
- A list of all of her previous surgeries, including the date, hospital, and surgeon; and
- Forms for each of her physicians on which she would list questions or concerns that she wanted to discuss on her next visit. Each form also included a location for her to enter the physician's responses. An example of this type of form is shown in Figure 4.12.

This approach worked very well for the client. Having one location with all of her medical information allowed her to quickly answer any questions that might come up about her medical care. If one of her physicians asked her what medications she was taking or who she was seeing for another aspect of her care, she had all of the details available. In fact, it worked so well for her that when her husband had an emergency surgery, she also included a section for his medical information in her organizer.

Medical Log for Dr. _____		
Date	**Questions**	**Notes From Office Visit**

Figure 4.12. Medical log, as used in Case D.

Doing Laundry. Another item we worked on during the first few weeks of treatment was getting the client to remember when there was laundry in progress. She often would start a load of laundry and then forget about it and leave it in the washing machine for days. The same thing would happen with the dryer. The solution to this was a simple placard that read "Laundry in Progress." I instructed her to post the placard in her kitchen where she would frequently encounter it whenever she started a load of laundry. This approach was simple but effective. Once she started using the placard she never reported another instance of forgetting about her laundry.

By the end of the first 4 weeks the client was no longer missing appointments and was consistently picking up her daughter from after-school activities. She was using the medical information section in her organizer effectively and no longer left laundry in the washer/dryer.

Revised Short-Term Goals (Weeks 5–10)

Building on the successful outcomes from the first 4 weeks of treatment, it was now time to begin working on more complex tasks. Although the laundry placard worked well once the laundry was in progress, getting it started was another issue. The client had great difficulty structuring her time throughout the week to allow for completion of routine household chores, including laundry and many other things. She also was easily confused about payment of bills and continued to accumulate late fees. During Weeks 5 through 10 we agreed to focus on the following items:

- Completing weekly home management tasks
- Development and use of an organized file system to track financial and other personal records.

Performing Weekly Home Management Tasks. One of the aspects of the client's brain injury was that she lost the ability to organize the tasks that she needed to complete each week into a manageable structure. She had no problems thinking of things that she needed to do but was unable to prioritize them. As a result, she would become frustrated and overwhelmed and would accomplish virtually nothing.

The client and I sat down and compiled a list of all of the routine household chores that she needed to complete each week, such as watering plants, vacuuming, and cleaning bathrooms. We generated a weekly checklist for all of her household chores. I knew from my experience with similar clients that this client's difficulties with initiation would prevent her from completing the items on the checklist unless specific times for each task were assigned. However, due to her varying appointment schedule, it was not practical to assign a consistent day and time each week for each task. For instance, she could not plan to water the plants each Monday at 10:00 a.m. because on some weeks she might have a doctor's appointment at that time. During the first 4 weeks of treatment, we had started a routine in which each Sunday evening the client and her daughter would meet and go through her appointments for the week and make sure they were listed in her personal organizer. This established routine provided the perfect opportunity to also go through the weekly checklist and assign specific times for each of the tasks.

This approach worked very well. Even in the first week of using it the client was able to complete nearly all of her weekly tasks.

Making an Organized File System. The client was consistently receiving late notices and getting phone calls regarding nonpayment of bills. To help her with this, I needed to understand the details of how she was attempting to keep track of her finances. I could not do this without going to her home and seeing for myself how things were organized. As I suspected, there were problems.

Upon entering her home office it was clear that things were in disarray. I asked her to guide me through her filing system, and it became apparent that she did not have one. She did have file cabinets and folders, but the records in them were not organized in any particular manner. Most folders contained information on multiple, unrelated topics. It was nearly impossible to locate a particular item such as last month's water bill or bank statement.

We emptied out all the file drawers and sorted through each folder. While doing so we found some of the bills the client thought she had already paid. Some contained checks made out for payment, but they had never been mailed. There was also a lot of junk mail that should have been discarded but instead ended up in various folders. I worked with the client to sort through the folders and keep only the important documents. We organized her file system to contain only a few general headings, such as utilities, cars, insurance, and medical, and a file folder was designated for each bill or topic.

Once her existing files were organized, we then worked out a system for tracking and filing new bills, account statements, and other records. We designated a plastic box on her office desk where all incoming bills would be placed. Upon receipt of a bill, the client was instructed to review the bill for accuracy and then write the due date on the outside of the envelope that it came in. She would then put the bill back inside that envelope and place it in the box along with any other bills that had arrived that week. The next step was to add "Pay Bills" to the weekly checklist. Following the procedure discussed above, each Sunday evening she would assign a time during the coming week when she would pay any bills that were due. The final step was to make the bill payment tracking form shown in Figure 4.13. All of her

Bill Payments	Due	Jan	Feb	Mar	Apr	May	Jun	Jul	Aug	Sept	Oct	Nov	Dec
Mortgage	1st												
St. Joe's Medical	1st												
Electricity	8th												
Water	12th												
Gas	15th												
Cable	15th												
Phone	15th												
Credit Card	21st												
Car Payment	21st												
Car Insurance													
Homeowners Association													

Figure 4.13. Bill-paying form, as used in Case D.

monthly bills were listed, along with their due dates on the form. Extra space was provided for any new or unexpected bills. The client was instructed to place a checkmark in the corresponding month only after the payment had been placed in the mail.

At weekly therapy sessions we monitored her bill-paying compliance over the next month by having her husband double check the payment of all bills. This structured approach worked very well, and within 1 month she was independent with this task.

Revised Short-Term Goals (Weeks 11–14)

By the end of 10 weeks the client was using her personal organizer to effectively structure her daily activities. She was no longer missing appointments, she was able to pay bills on time, and she was completing all of the weekly household chores on her checklist. At this point, she was ready to move on to more complicated duties. She was very motivated to be independent with meal planning, grocery shopping, and meal preparation, and we agreed that this would be the focus for the last few weeks of treatment.

During our next therapy session I started by asking the client about the foods she would typically prepare for family meals. We made the menu-planning list shown in Figure 4.14 and divided it into main dishes and side dishes. The only purpose of this list was to help her with her problem of not being able to think of what to make for dinner. By having the list available, she was able to select main and side dishes in many combinations. We added "Meal Planning" to her weekly checklist, and each Sunday evening after entering all appointments and household chores, she would then plan meals for the week. Armed with the menu-planning list, she was able to select meals for several nights each week, starting with 3 nights and eventually achieving her goal of 5 nights. She would write the menu for each meal in her personal organizer on the day she planned to make it and would make a note in the time slot when she would need to begin preparing the meal.

Once she had planned the meals for the upcoming week, the next step was to make sure that all the necessary ingredients were available. We went through each item on the menu-planning list and made a generic grocery list of all of the primary ingredients (Figure 4.15). Each week she would make a copy of this list and circle the items she needed to purchase, using the space at the bottom of the list for additional items. On Sunday evenings after planning the meals for the week, she would go through her kitchen and determine what she needed to include on the grocery list. She also

MAIN DISHES	SIDE DISHES
☐ Pork chops	☐ Mashed potatoes
☐ Chicken	☐ Red potatoes
☐ Hamburgers	☐ Baked potatoes
☐ Steak	☐ Rice
☐ Hot dogs	
☐ Fish	
☐ Spaghetti	☐ Broccoli with cheese
☐ Tacos	☐ Cucumbers
☐ Tostadas	☐ Sliced tomatoes
☐ Meat loaf	☐ Corn
	☐ Green beans
	☐ Black-eyed peas
	☐ Spinach
	☐ Salsa
	☐ Salad
	☐ Potato salad
	☐ Bread

Figure 4.14. Menu-planning list, as used in Case D.

would schedule a time in her organizer to do the grocery shopping.

After her first week of using this system the client reported only one major problem. She had planned on preparing chicken one night for dinner. On Sunday evening she had checked and found chicken in the freezer, so she did not add it to her grocery list. Later in the week when it came time to prepare the meal, the chicken was still frozen and could not be used that day. To solve such problems, I instructed her to include a note in her organizer on the day before the planned meal if an ingredient needed to be taken out of the freezer to thaw. She would include such a note for any items that needed to be prepared ahead of time while planning meals each Sunday evening. By the end of 14 weeks, she was planning and preparing all family meals independently.

Summary

When I first started working with this client, she was very anxious and overwhelmed by the effect her brain injury was having on her ability to be what she considered to be a good wife and mother. By initially focusing the treatment on a few small items and then gradually building on them, we were able over the course of treatment to define effective compensations for her most

DAIRY	BREADS AND CEREALS
☐ Milk	☐ Rice
☐ Half & half	☐ Taco shells
☐ Eggs	☐ Bread
☐ Cheese	☐ Hot dog buns
☐ Yogurt	☐ Hamburger buns
☐ Cottage cheese	☐ Breakfast cereal
☐ Cream cheese	**PRODUCE**
CANNED ITEMS	☐ Lettuce
☐ Spinach	☐ Tomatoes
☐ Refried beans	☐ Cucumbers
☐ Green beans	☐ Bananas
☐ Ranch beans	☐ Zucchini
☐ Black-eyed peas	☐ Carrots
☐ Corn	☐ Potatoes
☐ Soup	☐ Broccoli
☐ Salsa	☐ Corn
☐ Spaghetti sauce	☐ Onions
MEATS	☐ Garlic
☐ Pork chops	☐ Chilies
☐ Hot dogs	☐ Cilantro
☐ Chicken	**CONDIMENTS**
☐ Hamburger	☐ Mayonnaise
☐ Steak	☐ Mustard
☐ Fish	☐ Ketchup
FROZEN	
☐ Ice cream	
☐ Spinach	

Figure 4.15. Generic grocery list, as used in Case D.

pressing problems. The positive feedback that she received from her family was a great motivator for her. She began to feel productive at home and regained her self-worth. I saw this client in the community approximately 1 year after I stopped treating her. She reported continued success using and building on the compensations that we defined.

Case Example E: Outpatient and Work Reentry

59-Year-Old Man, Self-Employed Salesman, With Brainstem CVA

Illustrated in this example:
- Use of a comprehensive organizer system
- Use of customized forms and checklists
- Cross-referencing of organizer sections
- Benefits of a strong support network

Initial Evaluation

This client was first evaluated 7 months after a brainstem stroke. At that time, he had returned to work but was concerned that his memory deficits and fatigue were affecting his job performance. He had the long-term goal of maintaining his employment as an independent salesman. He was a representative for 15 different medical equipment companies and serviced approximately 250 customers in 3 states. His job required him to plan customer visits, provide on-site equipment demonstrations, place new customer orders, and follow up on previously placed orders. He said that he had missed two important appointments within the past 2 weeks. One was a customer meeting in another city, and the other was an in-service for the staff at a rehabilitation center. He was unsure if there were other appointments that he had missed. He said that when he did remember appointments, he often arrived without the necessary items, such as price lists, equipment brochures, and handouts.

The client reported that he had already tried using an organizer on his own but was unsuccessful. For example, he had scheduled a meeting by recording the meeting time and the first name of the customer but omitted the location of the meeting and the customer's last name. He was extremely frustrated and embarrassed by this situation because he knew that he had missed the appointment but did not know who to call to apologize.

He also had difficulty organizing receipts for billing and reimbursement. As a salesman, his income was linked directly to his sales as reported in his billing records. His memory problems were having a definite impact on his income, and his wife was becoming frustrated with him because of it.

The following deficits were apparent during the initial evaluation:
- Reduced mental and physical stamina
- Decreased speed of information processing
- Moderate memory deficits
- Mildly impaired attention and concentration.

These deficits were consistent with the client's neuropsychological test results, which indicated moderate memory difficulties as well as difficulties with concentration and attention to detail. Despite these deficits, the following factors made this client a good candidate for treatment:
- A strong motivation to work
- A growing awareness of his deficits

- A willingness to use compensatory strategies
- A willingness to modify and limit his job responsibilities
- Strong support from his spouse.

Focus of Treatment

Because this client needed to keep track of a large amount of information, it was immediately clear that a comprehensive organizer system, including full-sized daily dated pages, customized forms and checklists, and a wristwatch with an hourly chime/alarm, would be required.

On initial review, the complexity of this client's job duties coupled with his deficits made the long-term goal of achieving work independence seem very difficult to attain. Because the client's wife had worked as his assistant for many years and had a good understanding of the operation of his business, it was apparent that she should be involved in all treatment sessions. Fortunately, she was willing and able to participate in defining and implementing the treatment plan. I arranged to meet with the client and his wife twice a week over a 3-month period.

Initial Short-Term Goals (Weeks 1–4)

During my second meeting with the client and his wife, three short-term goals were defined:
- Get to appointments on time
- Complete a daily list of phone calls
- Track receipts for billing.

These goals were designed to simultaneously address the client's urgent business needs and provide a foundation for personal organizer use. To reach these goals, the client would need to learn how to write effective notes in the daily pages, where to enter and retrieve information, and how to use a wristwatch with an alarm.

Keeping Appointments. To get to an appointment on time, the client needed to know the time and place of the appointment and with whom he was meeting. To keep it simple, other details, such as the purpose of the meeting, were not tracked as part of the initial short-term goal. My meetings with the client and his wife would begin with a review of the daily pages in his organizer. We would review each entry to ensure that it was entered at the correct place on the correct page and contained the customer's name and the location of the meeting. Initially, many errors were encountered. Using his wife as a source of reliable data, corrections were dictated to the client. Rather than simply pointing out mistakes, the client was required to make corrected entries in his organizer while both his wife and I were present.

Many of my clients benefit from using a wristwatch with an hourly chime and alarm to help them keep track of their daily schedule. This client required very little instruction with the use of the wristwatch and was able to quickly learn to use it to prompt him to review his organizer and remind him of upcoming appointments. Although he used the watch extensively, my involvement was limited to telling him which watch to purchase and providing him detailed instructions for using the alarm and hourly chime.

At each session, his ability to record appointments in the correct location within the organizer and get to appointments on time was summarized by calculating a percentage of compliance. Within 3 weeks, he was 100% successful with these tasks.

Tracking Phone Calls. Before seeking treatment, the client had attempted to make lists of phone calls that he should make each day. These lists were very disorganized. They were kept in various locations (e.g., on sticky notes, on various slips of paper, in numerous locations in his organizer), and no system for ensuring that he actually made the calls was in place. I approached this problem by defining a location in his daily pages where all phone calls to be made that day would be listed. When calls were completed, they would be checked off the list. If for some reason a call was not made, it would be transferred to the list for the following day. Each evening he would review the list with his wife to ensure that all calls were either completed or moved to the next day. Again, his percentage of compliance was tracked, and within 1 month he reached a point at which he rarely made mistakes (more than 98% compliance). It is important to note that at this point we were not tracking the details of each call, only his ability to complete the call.

Managing Receipts. As with the phone calls, this client had no consistent place for keeping his billing receipts. At the end of the week he would have to search his car, all of his jackets, numerous customer files, and so forth to look for receipts. My approach was to provide a plastic pouch in his organizer where he would place all of his receipts. This approach worked well, and within the first week of treatment he was keeping track of his receipts with virtually no mistakes.

During the first month of treatment while focusing on the above-mentioned goals, I had the opportunity to learn some of the details of his business. As I learned more, it became clear that detailed forms and checklists would need to be developed to help him keep track of the content of the phone calls and appointments he had with customers.

Revised Short-Term Goals (Weeks 5–10)

By Week 5 the client was able to consistently get to appointments on time but was having difficulty recalling the content of his meetings and remembering to follow up on the details. Building on the foundation set by the initial goals, the following short-term goals were designed to help him with these problems:

- Keeping track of details of each appointment and phone call
- Bringing all of the necessary items to appointments.

Keeping Track of Details. During the first 4 weeks of treatment, the client began taking notes when talking with customers. Unfortunately, his notes were so disorganized that they were useless. He frequently left out pertinent information and did not keep the notes in any particular order. Furthermore, he was not consistent in his note taking. Sometimes he took notes, and other times he did not. He tended to keep his notes in chronological order on the daily pages and thus could not use them to quickly review past discussions with particular customers. His notes provided no framework for fulfilling customer requests. It was evident that he needed a well-organized tracking system for his interactions with each customer.

My first step was to figure out in detail what information the client needed to track. A thorough understanding of his business was needed and, fortunately, the client and his wife were able to help me with that during the first 4 weeks of treatment. In his business of selling medical equipment he needed to provide demonstration equipment and product brochures to all of his customers. Keeping track of those items was a major problem for him. In one instance he loaned a customer a demonstration electric wheelchair worth several thousand dollars but was unable to recall which customer he had left it with. Many times he would forget to bring updated brochures on customer visits, which would result in lost sales. Sometimes his customers would request a specific product or information, and he would forget to bring it on his next visit. All of these things made it very difficult for him to make a living in sales.

Using my knowledge of his business needs, I developed the customer form shown in Figure 4.16. The purpose of this form was to provide a single place for the client to record all of his interactions with a particular customer. Besides the customer's name, address, and phone number, the form had locations to record demonstration equipment and brochures (binders) given to the customer. A space also was provided to list important personnel contacts within the company. The main body of the customer form was used to record in chronological order all of the client's discussions with his customer. Columns for recording the date, contact person, and details of the discussion were provided.

To effectively use the customer forms, the client first needed to have the correct form with him whenever he would talk with a particular customer and also needed to learn to make meaningful entries on the form during the conversation. In this case, the client had 250 customers, making it unfeasible to carry all of the customer forms with him in his organizer. We decided to keep the forms in notebooks arranged by territory in the client's office. A section within the organizer was created to provide a place for the customer forms needed for the current day. Each evening the client and his wife would review the past day's activities and also the upcoming day's schedule. The customer forms for the past day would be returned to the office notebooks, and those for the next day were placed in the organizer. As the forms were reviewed, the notes would be checked for accuracy. Any corrections or additions to the notes would be made by the client under the direction of his wife. In this manner, his note taking gradually improved.

To effectively use the customer forms, the client needed to follow through on the actions discussed with the customer. Cross-referencing between the customer forms and daily pages was necessary. If the client agreed to a future meeting with a customer and recorded it on the customer form, that information would need to be transferred to the daily pages. Each evening with his wife, and also during each treatment session, the customer forms were carefully reviewed to ensure that all appointments and other commitments (e.g., product orders, returns, billing questions) that required action by the client were transferred to the appropriate sections of the organizer (e.g., daily pages, to-do lists, other forms) so that they would not be forgotten.

The client's progress with using the customer forms was tracked weekly by calculating his percentage of compliance with having the correct forms with him each day and with cross-referencing to the different sections of his organizer. Within 2 weeks this client was independent with keeping the correct customer forms in his organizer. After 6 weeks (Week 10 of the treatment), his note taking and cross-referencing reached a level of 80% compliance. His wife continued to work with him in this area, and he continued to improve as we moved on to new goals.

Bringing Items to Appointments. Within the first week of using the customer forms it became clear that the client would need an additional method of organizing

| Equipment _____ | Binder # given _____ |
| Date _____ |

Equipment _____

_____

Customer _____

Address _____

Phone _____

Binder # given _____

Date _____

Key Contacts _____

_____

_____

Date	Contact	Notes (Products discussed, decisions, interests, etc.)

Figure 4.16. Example customer form, as used in Case E.

his daily sales calls. As mentioned earlier, he would commonly forget to bring brochures, catalogs, and demonstration products on his customer visits. The client would typically visit 4 or 5 different customers each day. This meant that each day his organizer would contain 4 or 5 different customer forms, each with several actions that he needed to address. He would often become confused and forget to complete many of the items on the customer forms. He needed a place to summarize on 1 page all of his customer meetings for the day.

The sales call checklist shown in Figure 4.17 was developed to help him with these problems. This checklist included a section for him to list each customer he planned on visiting that day and summarize the objectives of each meeting. Each evening he and his wife would review the daily pages in his organizer to make a list of the customers that he planned to visit the next day. He would then retrieve their customer forms from the notebooks in his office and transfer the actions from each customer form to the sales call checklist objectives column. Then, using the objectives as a guide, he would gather all needed literature (e.g., brochures, catalogs, price lists) and products and place them in his van for the next day's visits. The sales call checklist was then placed in his organizer next to the daily page for the following day.

SALES CALLS

Make a list of all customers you intend to call on.
Date _____

Customer
Objectives

_____
_____
_____
_____
_____
_____
_____
_____
_____
_____
_____
_____
_____
_____
_____
_____
_____
_____
_____

- Pull all customer sheets and review (any products they are interested in, etc.).
- Gather literature about specific product.
    - Catalog
    - Price List
    - Selling Sheets
- Put products in the van.
- Bring organizer with you.
- Pull customer sheet from organizer to write on while you are with the customer.

Figure 4.17. Example sales call checklist, as used in Case E.

The client's progress with using the sales call checklist was tracked weekly by calculating his percentage of compliance with having the correct products and literature with him on each customer visit. After 4 weeks (Week 8 of the treatment), he reached 95% compliance with these tasks. At that point we quit monitoring his compliance in this area, but his wife continued to work with him to reach 100%.

Revised Short-Term Goals (Weeks 11–14)

By the end of Week 10 in the treatment plan, the client was consistently attending customer meetings and following through on action items. He was able to coordinate activities with his customers on a daily basis. With

this under control, the emphasis of the treatment plan changed to long-term planning of customer visits.

Planning Customer Visits. The client's business required him to service 250 customers in 3 states. Once he scheduled an appointment with a customer, he was able to follow through with minimal supervision. However, planning for visits to other states was difficult. He often could not remember when he had last visited customers out of his local area. This information was on his customer forms, but he needed a convenient method of reviewing it without thumbing through the 250 customer forms.

To solve this problem, a master customer list was developed for each of his sales territories. This was a simple list of the account names and contact dates as shown in Figure 4.18. Each time he would visit or call a customer he would record the contact date on the list and indicate whether it was a personal visit or phone call. By reviewing this list on a weekly basis, he was able to quickly determine when he needed to schedule his next trip to outlying territories.

Additional forms and checklists were developed for the client to use when planning training at customer facilities and for tracking equipment orders (Figures 4.19 and 4.20). It is important to note that development of forms and checklists is a trial-and-error process in which many revisions are made before a final version is completed.

Summary

When I first started working with this client, our long-term goal was for him to perform his job at a level com-parable to his prestroke abilities. As an independent salesperson he had responsibility for all aspects of his business. Even though his deficits were moderate, he required a comprehensive system because of the complexity of his job duties. To reach his final goal, a series of achievable short-term goals was used. I spent a large portion of my time with him learning the details of his business so that I could adapt an organizer system to meet his needs.

It is now more than 6 years after treatment, and the client is continuing to run his business. He does, however, still require assistance from his wife. She continues to meet with him each day to review his schedule, assist with ordering products, and help organize catalogs for customer visits. Both the client and his wife have expressed to me that they could not have continued to operate their business without the tools we developed to compensate for his deficits.

MASTER CUSTOMER LIST

Territory _____

Account Name	Contact Date				

Figure 4.18. Form used to track all customers, as used in Case E.

IN-SERVICES

- Call contact person to set up an in-service. Make a note of contact person's:

  Name _____

  Phone number_____

- Dealer involved _____

- Get directions if needed _____

  _____

  _____

- Decide with them what product you will feature _____

  _____

  _____

- Set a time and date_____

- If agreeing to provide food, make a note of this.

- Put this appointment in your organizer.

- Put a note in your organizer approximately 1 week prior to in-service to phone and confirm appointment. Refer to date of in-service in this note.

- Place this sheet of paper on the day before the in-service.

- Gather the product to feature and load in van.

- Gather all needed literature and put in van.

- Put all freebies in van if bringing any.

- Arrange for food if agreed on.

Figure 4.19. Checklist for on-site training, as used in Case E.

DEMO EQUIPMENT ORDERED

Order Date	Manufacturer	Equipment—Serial Number	Customer/Phone	Expected Date	Date Received

Figure 4.20. Form to track equipment orders, as used in Case E.

Summary

The case studies provided in this chapter are based on real clients that I have worked with over the past 15 years. I selected them to illustrate the wide range of memory compensation tools and techniques that can be applied in working with clients in a variety of stages of their rehabilitation. Memory problems have a profound effect on the quality of life of clients, their families, and loved ones. It is my hope that you, the reader, will be able to take some of the techniques I have described in this book and adapt them to your clients' needs to improve their quality of life.

Reference

Wilson, B., Cockburn, J., Baddeley, A., Hiorns, R., Smith, P., Ivani-Chalian, R., et al. (1989). *Rivermead Behavioural Memory Test* (RMBT). Titchfield, UK: Thames Valley Test Company.

Suggested Reading

D'Esposito, M., & Alexander, M. P. (1995). The clinical profiles, recovery, and rehabilitation of memory disorders. *NeuroRehabilitation, 5,* 141–159.

Dirette, D. (2004). A comparison of attention, processing, and strategy use by adults with and without acquired brain injuries. *Brain Injury, 18,* 1219–1227.

Dixon, R. A., deFrias, C. M., & Backman, L. (2001). Characteristics of self-reported memory compensation in older adults. *Journal of Experimental Neuropsychology, 23,* 650–661.

Doornheim, K., & DeHaan, E. H. F. (1998). Cognitive training for memory deficits in stroke patients. *Neuropsychological Rehabilitation, 8,* 393–400.

Goldstein, G., Ryan, C., Turner, S. M., Kanagy, M., Barry, K., & Kelly, L. (1985). Three methods of memory training for severely amnesic patients. *Behavior Modification, 9,* 357–374.

Hart, T., O'Neil-Pirozzi, T., & Morita, C. (2003). Clinical expectations for portable electronic devices as cognitive–behavioural orthoses in traumatic brain injury rehabilitation. *Brain Injury, 17,* 401–411.

Johansson, U., & Bernspang, B. (2003). Life satisfaction related to work re-entry after brain injury: A longitudinal study. *Brain Injury, 17,* 991–1002.

Katz, N., Fleming, J., Keren, N., Lightbody, S., & Hartman-Maeir, A. (2002). Unawareness and/or denial of disability: Implications for occupational therapy intervention. *Canadian Journal of Occupational Therapy, 69,* 281–292.

Kim, H. J., Burke, D. T., Dowds, Jr., M. M., Robinson Boone, K. A., & Park, G. J. (2000). Electronic memory aids for outpatient brain injury: Follow-up findings. *Brain Injury, 14,* 187–196.

Manchester, D., Priestley, N., & Jackson, H. (2004). The assessment of executive functions: Coming out of the office. *Brain Injury, 18,* 1067–1081.

O'Carroll, R. E., Russell, H. H., Lawrie, S. M., & Johnstone, E. C. (1999). Errorless learning and the cognitive rehabilitation of memory-impaired schizophrenic patients. *Psychological Medicine, 29,* 105–112.

Power, P. W., & Hershenson, D. B. (2003). Work adjustment and readjustment of persons with mid-career onset traumatic brain injury. *Brain Injury, 17,* 1021–1034.

Prigatano, G., Fordyce, D., Zeiner, H., Roueche, J., Pepping, M., & Wood, B. (1984). Neuropsychological rehabilitation after closed-head injury in young adults. *Journal of Neurology, Neurosurgery, and Psychiatry, 47,* 505–513.

Roche, N. L., Fleming, J. M., & Shum, D. H. K. (2002). Self-awareness of prospective memory failure in adults with traumatic brain injury. *Brain Injury, 16,* 931–945.

Squires, E. J., Hunkin, N. M., & Parkin, A. J. (1996). Memory notebook training in a case of severe amnesia: Generalising from paired associate learning to real life. *Neuropsychological Rehabilitation, 6*(1), 55–65.

Tate, R. L. (1997). Beyond one-bun, two-shoe: Recent advances in the psychological rehabilitation of memory disorders after acquired brain injury. *Brian Injury, 11,* 907–918.

Thompson, P. J. (1991). Memory function in patients with epilepsy. *Advances in Neurology, 55,* 369–384.

Wilson, B. A., Baddeley, A. D., Evans, J. J., & Shiel, A. (1994). Errorless learning in the rehabilitation of memory impaired people. *Neuropsychological Rehabilitation, 4,* 307–326.

Zangwill, O. L. (1947). Psychological aspects of rehabilitation in cases of brain injury. *British Journal of Psychology, 37,* 60–69.

Zencius, A., Wesolowski, M. D., & Burke, W. H. (1990). A comparison of four memory strategies with traumatically brain-injured clients. *Brain Injury, 4,* 33–38.

Index

Note: Entries in *italic* refer to figures

About the Author

Susan K. Kime, OTR/L, received her BA in occupational therapy from the College of St. Catherine in St. Paul, Minnesota. During the 25 years since receiving her degree she has worked extensively with clients with brain injury in a wide variety of treatment settings from intensive care through outpatient rehabilitation. She currently has a private practice in Phoenix, Arizona, where she focuses on developing and implementing strategies to compensate for residual memory and cognitive deficits with clients with brain injury or other neurological impairment. She has taught courses and lectured in the United States, Sweden, and England. Articles on her work have been published in the journals *Brain Injury* and *NeuroRehabilitation*.